Emna Marmech

Pneumothorax during the first 24 hours of life:

Emna Marmech

Pneumothorax during the first 24 hours of life:

Risk factors and management

ScienciaScripts

Cover image: www.ingimage.com

This book is a translation from the original published under ISBN 978-620-6-71715-7.

Publisher:
Sciencia Scripts
is a trademark of
Dodo Books Indian Ocean Ltd. and OmniScriptum S.R.L publishing group

120 High Road, East Finchley, London, N2 9ED, United Kingdom
Str. Armeneasca 28/1, office 1, Chisinau MD-2012, Republic of Moldova, Europe
Managing Directors: Ieva Konstantinova, Victoria Ursu
info@omniscriptum.com

Printed at: see last page
ISBN: 978-620-8-53487-5

Contents

1 INTRODUCTION

Pneumothorax (PNO) is a condition frequently encountered in neonatology. Its incidence is difficult to determine, as it may go unnoticed. However, it is more common in newborns (1 - 2%) than in older children (1.2 - 28 per 100,000), and can affect up to 30% of mechanically ventilated newborns.

Pneumothorax can occur in spontaneously ventilated newborns; this is spontaneous PNO, which occurs either on healthy lung parenchyma, and is referred to as primary spontaneous PNO, or on underlying lung pathology, and is referred to as secondary spontaneous PNO.

It is a diagnostic and therapeutic emergency that can lead to life-threatening respiratory and circulatory failure.

Clinical diagnosis is sometimes difficult. Diagnostic certainty is based on a chest x-ray. It involves a pleural detachment of varying severity.

Management, which must be immediate, vigorous and controlled in order to avoid the complications of hypoxaemia, hypercapnia and abnormal venous return, depends on the size of the effusion and varies according to the habits of the medical care team, given the absence of recommendations for the use of BNP during the neonatal period.

In Tunisia, few studies have been carried out to determine the prevalence, risk factors, progression and management of this condition during the neonatal period.

With this in mind, the aim of this study is to determine the risk factors for pneumothorax occurring during the first 24 hours of life in neonates admitted to the neonatal intensive care unit, and to outline the different management methods.

2 PATIENTS AND METHODS

I. Scope of the study :

Our study was carried out in the neonatology and neonatal intensive care unit of the Tunis Maternity and Neonatology Centre (CMNT), a level III neonatal care unit. The gynaecology and obstetrics departments of the CMNT are referral departments for high-risk pregnancies.

Part of the department's activity is managed in the nurseries. Children in nurseries in obstetrics sectors are separated from their mothers and do not benefit from specialist paediatric supervision outside paediatricians' hours of presence.

The criteria for admission to the nurseries included :

- Asymptomatic newborns with suspected maternal-tetal infection
- Newborns of diabetic mothers requiring blood glucose monitoring
- Newborns with intrauterine growth retardation, oligohydramnios, hydramnios, malformations requiring outpatient investigations.
- Newborns whose mothers are taking medication that may interfere with glycaemic control
- Newborns whose mothers have thrombocytopenia
- Asymptomatic premature newborns between 35 and 37 days' gestation
- Newborns with imperfect adaptation to life outside the womb who required a short resuscitation period using positive pressure ventilation (PPV) with good recovery.

Secondary hospitalisation may be necessary.

Admission to the department's intensive care unit was indicated for all symptomatic neonates. The reasons for admission were broad, including neonatal respiratory distress in term or near-term newborns not improving after 2 hours in Hood, the possibility of disease or malformation likely to cause sudden decompensation (cardiac, metabolic, etc.), premature births <34 SA, perinatal asphyxia....

II. Methods :

This is a retrospective, descriptive and analytical study involving 96 children admitted to the CMNT neonatology and neonatal intensive care unit over a two-year period from 1 November 2014 to 31 October 2016.

II.1 1 Inclusion criteria :

Our study consisted of recruiting newborn infants (NN) hospitalised in the department during the chosen period, who had presented with a pneumothorax during the first 24 hours of life and who had received care in the neonatal medicine and intensive care unit.

Patients were recruited in the delivery room. All newborns admitted to the department were assessed by the medical team present.

In our study, we included all newborns born at the CMNT and hospitalised in the department during the study period with a gestational age (GA) between 27 and 42 completed weeks of amenorrhoea (SA) and a birth weight (BW) >700 grams.

The diagnosis of PNO was suspected on clinical grounds and confirmed by chest X-ray:

J Clinical criteria: Respiratory distress

cyanosis; desaturation; distension of a hemi thorax; abolition of vesicular murmurs, A

subcutaneous emphysema

J Radiological criteria: well-defined hyperclarity with disappearance of lung parenchyma

The control population was chosen by chance and included newborns in respiratory distress whose births immediately followed or preceded the cases.

II.2 2 Exclusion criteria :

We have excluded :

J newborn babies transferred after birth to the Maternity Centre and taken into secondary care in the department (out-born).

J Newborns with PNO beyond the ^{24th} hour of life.

J Newborns of less than 27 weeks' gestation and/or with a PN <700 grams, for whom a collegial decision has been taken to refrain from resuscitation (DNR: do not rescuscitate), although support is provided (palliative) including rewarming and tube feeding.This attitude has not been pragmatic, and in some cases, relentless treatment has been adopted for certain newborns from so-called "precious" pregnancies, particularly when the chances of subsequent procreation are compromised (elderly mother, serious maternal pathology, parental sterility, haemostasis hysterectomy, etc.).

II.3 3 Data collection :

The information relating to each observation was recorded on an individual form from the medical records. (Appendix 1)

The form included various variables relating to maternal characteristics, the course of the pregnancy (pregnancy-related pathology, antenatal corticosteroid therapy, etc.), the course of the perinatal period, the characteristics of the NN and the circumstances in which the PNO occurred, its characteristics, as well as the therapeutic management and progress.

- Maternal characteristics :

Data on the mother were collected, specifying maternal age, geographical origin, occupation, level of education, consanguinity, parity, and medical history, in particular diabetes and arterial hypertension. We specified whether the mother had received antenatal corticosteroids in the case of premature delivery, and the antibiotic therapy prescribed during the 4 hours preceding delivery in the case of:

- Premature rupture of the membranes, defined as a rupture of the water sac for more than 12 hours before the start of labour.
- Isolated fever (over 38°C)
- chorioamniotitis
- urinary tract infection or any other infection.
- **The course of pregnancy :**

Certain information has been clarified:

^ Pregnancy monitoring: a pregnancy is considered to be monitored if the number of prenatal consultations is at least equal to 4, regularly distributed throughout the gestation period, with a minimum number of antenatal ultrasounds of 3.

^ The nature of chronic and associated pathologies

 pregnancy (toxaemia, gestational diabetes, etc.) and the treatment being used.

^ If it was an induced pregnancy, the procreation methods were specified.

^ The modalities of antenatal corticosteroid therapy: the number of doses received, the nature of the molecule administered (Dexamethasone or Bethamethasone) as well as the delay in its administration before delivery (less or more than 4 hours).the two molecules currently used are :

> Bethamethasone (Celestene): 12 mg/d as a single IM dose, 2 days in a row.

> Dexamethasone (Soludecadron): 6 mg*2/d IM, 2 days in a row; this drug is used in almost all cases at the CMNT; a course of treatment is considered complete if 12 mg IM is administered twice a day.

A course of treatment is said to be incomplete if a single dose has been administered more than 4 hours before delivery.

- Giving birth :

We specified the mode of delivery: vaginal delivery (VBD), with or without manoeuvres, or caesarean section. The timing of the caesarean section before or during labour was determined, as well as the reason for this indication: maternal and/or freight rescue.

- **Newborn babies :**

We specified gestational age, sex, Apgar score and birth measurements. We specified the time and reason for admission.

- **Diagnosis of pneumothorax :**

The positive diagnosis of PNO was made in the majority of cases on the chest X-ray. The chest X-ray was used to classify the PNO according to its severity as a simple detachment, a moderate PNO or a severe PNO. The latter was performed either systematically in all cases of neonatal respiratory distress or in all mechanically ventilated neonates, or when the clinical situation worsened. The radiological appearance corresponded to the presence or combination of the following images: Hyperclarity with disappearance of the pulmonary parenchyma on the affected side; Reduction or absence of pulmonary vascularisation ; Increase in the volume of the affected hemi thorax; Enlargement of the intercostal spaces; Flattening of the diaphragmatic dome on the affected side; Deviation of the mediastinum and/or Creur and/or trachea with reduction in the volume of the healthy lung; Narrow cardiac silhouette.

The PNO was considered as :

z Minimal if the detachment was less than 20 - 25% of the total lung volume

z Moderate if the detachment was between 25% and 40% of the total lung volume

J Severe if the detachment was greater than 40% of the total lung volume

PNO is classified as spontaneous PNO if the newborn has not received a PPV. It is termed primary or idiopathic spontaneous PNO if it occurs in healthy lung parenchyma and secondary spontaneous PNO if it occurs in underlying lung pathology.

In cases of immediately suffocating PNO, the diagnosis was suspected on physical examination (worsening of a previously well-controlled DRNN not responding to resuscitation, whether or not associated with auscultatory asymmetry; absence of chest indrawing on application of a PPV, reduction or abolition of the vesicular murmur), and management was initiated without waiting for the radiograph to be taken.

- Comprehensive care :

In addition to the care common to all newborns (warming, incubation, conditioning, monitoring, cord care, eye drops, vitamin K injections, venous access, etc.), certain treatments were administered depending on the GA and the initial condition of the patients, as well as any associated pathology:

J In cases of suspected maternal-fetal infection (MFI), antibiotic therapy for maternal-fetal use was initiated, combining betalactam antibiotics and aminoglycosides. This approach would be reviewed at a later date in the light of anamnestic, clinical, paraclinical and progressive data.

J Caffeine citrate was used prevent idiopathic apnoea of prematurity in newborns with GA<34SA. This treatment was administered as an initial loading dose of 20mg/kg on the first day in a single intravenous dose, followed by a maintenance dose of 5mg/kg/d.

We specified the timing, type and duration of invasive procedures such as intubation, placement of central venous catheters, exsufflation and chest drainage.

Below are the ventilatory supports adopted in our department:

(Appendix 4)

Table I: Ventilatory support the neonatal care unit

	Resources	Settings
Nasal CPAP	Infant Flow System Driver	s Flow 8l/mn s PEEP 5 to 6 cm of water s FiO2 for SpO2: 88-92% :AG<30SA/PN<1250gr 90-94% :AG>30SA /PN>1250gr
INSUREX	Exogenous surfactant: CUROSURF	Intra-tracheal: 100mg/kg
VC	Babylog 8000/Stephany (conventional mode)	VACI: s Flow 8l/mn s Pi:16-20cm H2O s PEP:3-5 cmH2O s Frequency:40-60cycles/mn s VT:4-6ml/kg s Minute volume:200-3000ml/kg/min s Ti as a function of PN -750-1000g:Ti=0,25-0,3 s -1000g-1500g: Ti=0,3s ->1500get>34 SA:Ti=0,35s ->34 SA:Ti=0,35-0,4s
OHF	Medis/Stephany sensor (OHF mode)	s Flow rate 20l/mn s Ti=0.5 sec s MAP>2 compared to MAP on Babylog (unless emphysema, decrease by 2) s If OHF from the outset:MAP =10-12 cmH2O:increase by 1 every 5 minutes, but clear plateau at 15 without exceeding 20 (goal FIO2>35%) except in exceptional cases s Frequency:15Hz for premature babies: if compliance is poor, reduce by 2-3 s Peak to Peak:start at 30-35 and adjust according to vibration and PCO2
NO	Nitrogen monoxide	s If NN term:10ppm up to 20ppm s If NN premature: 2ppm and increase 2ppm every 10mn to reach 5ppm maximum, exceptionally 10ppm s Stop: if methaemoglobin >5%.

The ventilatory management of our patients followed a pre-established protocol in our neonatal care unit (NICU).

The protocol is as follows:

Table II: Ventilation protocol in the neonatal care unit

Support	Indications
Nasal CPAP	In all cases of DRNN in premature infants with radiological alveolar syndrome, except where contraindicated ✓ From the outset: GA>30SA and/or PN<1000gr If 30 SA<AG<34SA with a 1000gr<PN<1250gr ✓ In the first 2 hours of life for: NN 30SA<AG<34SA and PN>1250gr if FiO2>30%. AG>34SA, if FiO2>40%.
INSUREX	✓ Straight away: GA<30SA and/or 750gr< PN<1250gr If PN<750gr jntubation-suffactant-conventional ventilation(CV) then extubation - CPAP,to be considered after 1 hour of CV. ✓ In the first 2 hours of life for NN of AG>30SA and/or PN>1500 gr, if FiO2>30%.
VC	After failure of 1я nCPAP

	✓ If AG<30SA (after administration of surfactant): FiO2>50%. ✓ If AG :30-34SA :FiO2>65% ✓ If GA> 34 SA; FiO2>65% and PCO2>60mmHg ✓ Recurrent apnoea
OHF	✓ PN<1500gr under IACV:if FiO2>70% and MAP>9mmHg and/or PCO2>60mmHg ✓ PN>1500gr,under IVAC:if FiO2>70% and/or MAP>12mmHg and/or PCO2>60mmHg
NO	✓ PAH: FiO2=100% and SaO<88% with PO2<50mmHg ✓ FiO2>50% and ultrasound data compatible with PAH

. NICU management of PNO :

The management of PNO depended on the severity and clinical tolerance and consisted either:

> A wait-and-see attitude: this consisted of putting the NN under hyperoxia with Fio2=100% in the case of minimal, non-symptomatic PNO requiring rigorous, close clinical and radiological monitoring

> Exsufflation with or without thoracic drainage. The exsufflation and drainage techniques are described in Appendices 2 and 3.

> Suspension of drainage with close and rigorous clinical and radiological monitoring was indicated in cases of minimal primary spontaneous PNO which had completely resolved after exsufflation with a stable haemodynamic and neurological state.

> Immediate chest drainage without exsufflation if the newborn is stable and has a moderate to large PNO.

> Mechanical ventilation was indicated for all neonates who had been drained. If a mechanical ventilation machine was not available, the newborn was placed in hyperoxia under CPAP.

> Treat newborns for FMD caused by atypical germs, particularly in cases of primary spontaneous PNO and in the presence of an infectious anamnesis

II.4 Statistical analysis :

Data processing and statistical analysis carried out using SPSS 19 software.

- Descriptive study :

- For qualitative variables, we calculated simple frequencies and relative frequencies (percentages).
- For qualitative variables, we calculated means, medians and standard deviations, and determined the range for quantitative variables.

- Analytical study :

- Comparisons of two means on independent series were carried out using the Student's t-test for independent series and, in the case of small numbers, the non-parametric Mann Withney test.

- Comparisons of two percentages on independent series were carried out using Pearson's chi2 test and, in the event of invalidity, Fisher's exact test.

- Identification of risk factors :

- Univariate study: The search for risk factors was carried out by calculating the Odds ratio, which represents the number of times by which the probability (risk) of an event (occurrence of PNO) is multiplied in case of exposure to a factor compared with non-exposure.

Multivariate study: In order to identify the risk factors independently linked to the event, we carried out a multivariate analysis using stepwise top-down logistic regression (at the first stage, we introduced all the factors with a "p" of 0.05 in the univariate analysis and those with a "p" of between 0.05 and 0.15, and from stage to stage we removed the factor with the least significant "p"). Multivariate analysis was used to calculate adjusted Odds Ratios, measuring the specific role of each factor.

The difference between two parameters is considered significant when the "p" significance level is less than 0.05.

II.5 Definitions :

- **Premature rupture of the membranes**

Premature rupture of the membranes is defined as a rupture of the amnion and chorion at the lower pole of the uterus before the onset of labour, and is considered to be a clear, abundant fluid discharge which occurs suddenly and repeatedly. Blood gas measurements could not be carried out in some cases due to lack of resources.

- **Apparent death :**

When the Apgar score at 1 minute of life is less than 3, the newborn is considered to be in a state of apparent death, reflecting a failure to adapt to life outside the womb. The clinical signs are: ineffective or absent respiratory movements: apnoea (or gasps) - heart rate < 60/min (or even heart rate 0)

-Intense, generalised cyanosis (and/or pallor)

- **Perinatal asphyxia :**

The diagnosis of APN was based on clinical and anamnestic elements (SFA, HRP, haemorrhagic placenta previa, T3 haemorrhage....) and an

Apgar score at 5th minute of less than 7/10. The

- **Maternal-frequent infection (MFI) :**

The diagnosis of maternal-fetal infection was suspected on the basis of a range of anamnestic (premature and/or prolonged rupture of membranes >12h, maternal fever, burning micturition, leucorrhoea, foul amniotic fluid, unexplained prematurity, unexplained AFS, maternal hyperleukocytosis, increased maternal CRP .), clinical, biological (hyperleukocytosis, thrombocytopenia, neutropenia, CRP >6mg/l) and confirmed by bacteriological data.

- **Hyaline membrane disease (HMD):**

The diagnosis of MMH was made on the basis of clinical and radiological criteria: it was a progressive onset of DRNN, with significant draught associated with a diffuse bilateral alveolar infiltrate and a decrease in lung volume.

- **Pulmonary arterial hypertension (PAH):**

The diagnosis of PAH was based on clinical and radiological criteria: severe DRNN with very high oxygen requirements; a difference between supraductal and subductal oxygen saturation > or = 10%; a newborn who worsens his cyanosis at the slightest stimulation; and a thirax radiograph showing clear lungs or a "clear" lung.

Slight parenchymal involvement contrasting with the severity of the clinical picture and the absence of a heart murmur. Confirmation by Doppler ultrasound was not possible.

- **Suffocating PNO:**

Suffocating or compressive pneumothorax occurs when an abnormal accumulation air between the two layers of the pleura causes suffocation by pressure on the lungs. Suffocating pneumothorax is characterised by pleural pressure above atmospheric pressure. It is life-threatening due to circulatory distress (gas tamponade).

- **N-CPAP (nasal continuous positive pressure) :**

Also known as nasal CPAP (nasal continuous positive airway pressure). PEEP is delivered via nasal devices to a spontaneously ventilating newborn. Nasal PEEP can be applied either with a nasal tube or with a device that uses flow acceleration to maintain positive pressure throughout the child's respiratory cycle (Infant Flow system).

- **VC: conventional ventilation**

In this type of ventilation, the ventilator generates cyclical variations in airway pressure, the maximum pressure of which is called the maximum inspiratory pressure (Pi max). This is the main ventilation technique used in neonates, and allows several ventilation modes, the two main ones being controlled ventilation and assisted or self-triggered ventilation.

- **VAC: controlled assisted ventilation :**

This mode is called assisted because the ventilator gives an insufflation each time the child makes a call and triggers the cycle, and controlled because if the child is not breathing, the machine delivers a minimum set by the operator.

- **VACI: intermittent controlled assisted ventilation :**

This mode is similar to CAV, the only difference being that the number of assisted cycles does not exceed the frequency set by the operator. If the child makes calls beyond the set frequency, the machine allows him to breathe spontaneously, but does not deliver insufflations.

- **OHF: High Frequency Oscillation :**

It uses small tidal volumes, often less than the dead space, and extremely fast frequencies (>5 Hz or five times the patient's natural frequency; 1 Hz = 60/min). There are several types:

- high-frequency flow interruption ventilation, often abbreviated VHF.

-High frequency oscillation ventilation (HFO): the tidal volume is actively produced by the back and forth movement a membrane or piston.

Our service uses the high-frequency flow interruption mode (Babylog 8000 HFVT).

II.6 Collection of bibliographical data

We used the Science direct and Pubmed websites to search for recent articles using the following key words validated on Pubmed: Pneumothorax - neonates - risk factors - respiratory distress - emergency.

This bibliography helped us to understand the work, particularly with regard to the methodology to be followed and the recording of results, and enabled us to compare our results with those of published series and to identify and comment on some of the study's biases.

No thesis on neonatal PNO has been published in the libraries of the 4 faculties of medicine.

II.7 Ethical considerations and conflicts of interest

We have no conflicts of interest in relation to this study.

A. CHARACTERISTICS OF THE STUDY POPULATION :

I. Global data :

During the period from 1st November 2014 to 31 October 2016, we recorded 28 800 live births at the Tunis Maternity and Neonatology Centre, including 5540 admissions to the neonatal intensive care unit. The reasons for hospitalisation varied between prematurity, infection, DRNN and other conditions.

Neonatal respiratory distress was the main reason for hospitalisation.

I.1 Incidence of PNO in the first 24 months of life

During the study period, we diagnosed 136 cases of pneumothorax, 104 of which were excluded from our study. The newborns excluded from our study were distributed as follows:

J 6 Cas de out born

J 10 cases in which the PN was less than 750g and/or the GA was less than 27 SA

J 88 cases of PNO occurring beyond 24 hours of life A total of **32 cases** were included in our study**.** The incidence of PNO occurring during the **first** 24 **hours of life was 1.1/1000 births.**

Sixty-four neonates admitted to hospital either before or immediately after the admission of the cases studied, and who had been admitted for NRD, were chosen as controls.

I.2 Prevalence of PNO compared to other DRNN :

DR, for all causes and all gestational ages, affected 6.4% of NV and accounted for 34% of ICU admissions (unpublished data).

The prevalence of neonatal PNO during neonatal respiratory distress was 5.4%.

PNO during the first 24 hours of life was diagnosed in 32 cases, i.e. a prevalence of 1.6% compared with all causes of DRNN.

II. Maternal characteristics :

II.1 1 Maternal age :

The average maternal age was 31.7 years, with extremes of 21 and 42 years.

The majority of the women were aged between 30 and 34.

years of age. Mothers aged over 35 accounted for 31.3% of cases. The distribution of parturients by age is summarised in Figure 2.

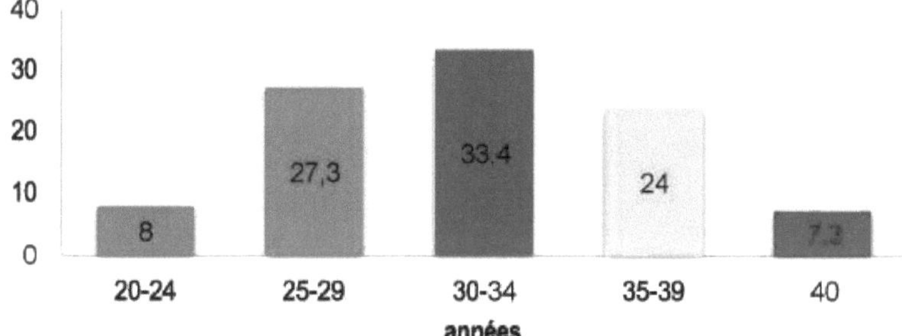

Figure 1: Age distribution of parturients

II.2 2 Other maternal characteristics :

More than two thirds of the parturients (69.3%) were housewives. In-utero transfers were noted in 6 cases.

A maternal pathology added to the pregnancy was found in 16.7% of parturients, with a particular predominance of chronic hypertension (6.7%), which combined with diabetes (4.7%) accounted for more than two-thirds of chronic maternal pathologies.

It should be noted that almost a third of parturients were primiparous and 41.3% of women were primigravida.

Parental consanguinity was noted in 12.8% of cases.

We noted a history of death in the siblings in 1 case at the age of 6 months. The chosen aetiology was metabolic disease.

There was no history of PNO in siblings or parents.

III. Characteristics of pregnancy and childbirth

III.1 Pregnancy :

- Pregnancy was spontaneous in 100% of cases
- Pregnancy monitoring was deemed to be compliant in 87.5% of cases.
- 2 cases of multiple pregnancy were recorded.
- Gestational toxaemia complicated 12.5% of pregnancies - Gestational diabetes during pregnancy was noted in 21.9% of cases
- Amniotic fluid was normal in 27

No cases of hydramnios were reported.

- 3 cases of placenta previa (9.6%) were reported.
- a single case of diaphragmatic hernia with pulmonary hypoplasia diagnosed antenatally was reported. Another case of renal agenesis in

the Potter sequence was noted (this is a series of characteristic malformations of the newborn following oligohydramnios).

Table III: Pregnancy characteristics

Pregnancy progress	Number	Percentage(%)
Compliant pregnancy monitoring	28	87,5
Monofetal pregnancy	30	93,8
RPM greater than 12H	4	12,5
Pregnancy toxaemia	4	12,5
Gestational diabetes	7	21,9
Oligohydramnios	5	15,6

III.2 Delivery characteristics :

> **Recording the RCF**

- The delivery was complicated by acute fretal distress in 6 newborns, a rate of 18.8%.

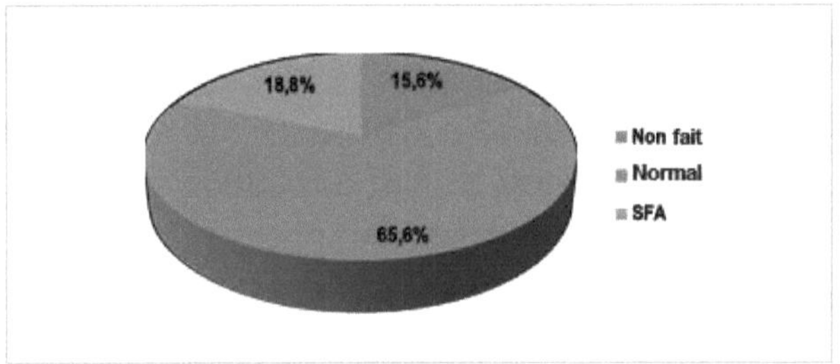

Figure 2: RCF recording

- Meconium amniotic fluid was found in 1 newborn, and 3 cases of stained amniotic fluid, representing 9.4% of newborns.
- There was only one case retroplacental haematoma.
- A cord circular was noted 3 cases, i.e. 9.4%.
- 5 newborns had a breech presentation (15.6%)
- **Delivery method :**
- The caesarean section rate (hot and cold) 59.4%. The caesarean section was performed as an emergency in 7 cases and was elective in 12 newborns, i.e. 60% of all caesarean sections and 37.5% of PNO cases.
- Instrumental delivery using Forceps was noted in 1 case. Delivery procedures are summarised in Figure 3

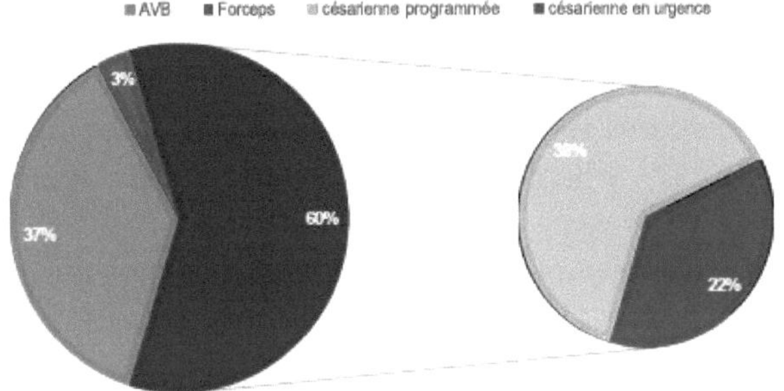

Figure 3: The different delivery methods

IV. Characteristics of newborn babies :

IV.1 Breakdown by gender :

The sex ratio (M/F) was 1.6. It was therefore predominantly male.

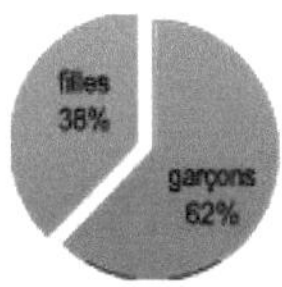

Figure 4: Breakdown by gender

IV.2 Distribution by birth weight :

The average birth weight was 2636g, with a minimum of 1150g and a maximum of 4360g. The very low birth weight population represented 15.6% of the study population. Figure 5 summarises the distribution of the population according to birth weight.

Figure 5: Breakdown by birth weight

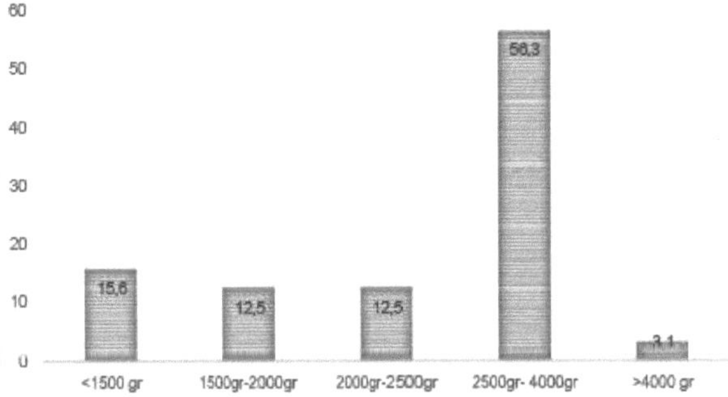

IV.3 Distribution according to gestational age :

-The mean GA in our series was 35.7 SA with extremes ranging from 28 to 41.3 SA.

- Half of the newborns were premature (GA < 37 SA), 25% of whom were very premature. Prematurity was spontaneous in 10 cases.
- No newborns were born post-term (GA> 42 SA)

Figure 6 summarises the distribution of the population by birth weight.

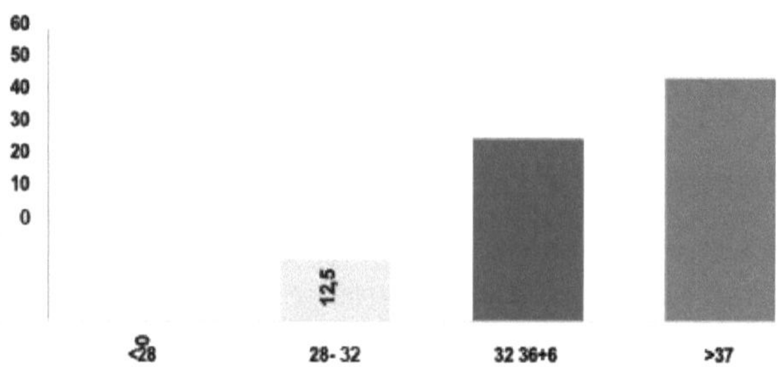

Figure 6 : Distribution according gestational age

IV.4 Condition of newborn babies in the delivery room :

- Two patients were born in a state of apparent death (Apgar at 1 min <3)
- an Apgar score<=7 at 5th minute was noted in 18.8% of newborn babies
- Mask ventilation in the delivery room was used in 12 neonates (37.5%).
- Eight newborns were intubated in the delivery room
- IUGR was observed in 2 cases

B.CHARACTERISTICS OF PNEUMOTHORAX

1. Overall analysis :

- The diagnosis of PNO was suspected clinically and confirmed by chest X-ray in 30 NN. In two cases, the PNO occurred immediately after birth: the diagnosis was suspected clinically in the presence of an apparent state of death that did not respond to resuscitation. An incidental finding of a PNO on the radiograph was reported in 7 cases: this was a minimal pleural detachment.
- The main manifestation of PNO was superficial polypnoea in 78% of

cases. The median respiratory rate was 75 cycles/min.

- The median Silverman score (SS) was 4 with extremes from zero to eight; signs of struggle were marked in 8 newborns, with a SS >4 (25%). The SS was minimal between 0 and 1 in 3 newborns, i.e. 9.4% of cases.

Cyanosis was noted in 59.4% of neonates, with extreme desaturation of up to 12%. SaO2 was not always mentioned given the often abrupt onset of PNO requiring urgent management.

- In 50% of cases, the PNO was diagnosed before H1 of life and in 25% of cases within the first 12 hours of life. Figures 7 and 8 show respectively the distribution of the time of onset of pneumothorax to gestational age and birth weight. All newborns with a birth weight >2500 had developed a PNO within the first hour of life. Figures 7 and 8 show the distribution of the time of onset of pneumothorax according to GA and birth weight.

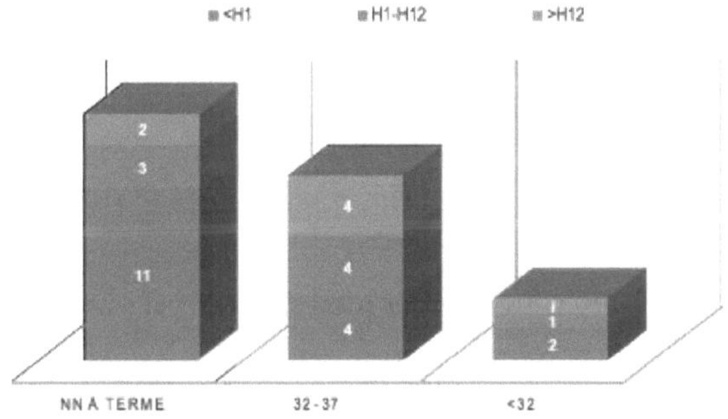

Figure 7: Time of onset of pneumothorax and gestational age

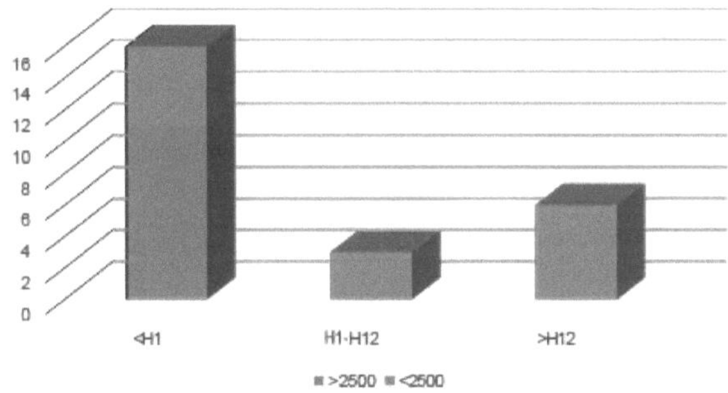

Figure 8: Distribution of pneumothorax according to birth weight and time of onset

- Signs of seriousness (haemodynamic or neurological disorders) were noted in 15 newborns, i.e. 46.8% of cases.
- The initial PNO was suffocating in 31.2% and minimal in 28.1%.
- PNO was associated with pneumo-mediastinum in 7 cases.
- The PNO was classified as spontaneous in 59.3% of cases

It was a primary spontaneous PNO in eight newborns (25%) where no associated cause was identified; and was a secondary spontaneous PNO in 34.3%. In term newborns, infectious alveolitis was the main aetiology associated with secondary spontaneous PNO, whereas in premature infants, hyaline membrane disease (HMD) was the main pathology found. Fig. 9 summarises GA classification of PNO.

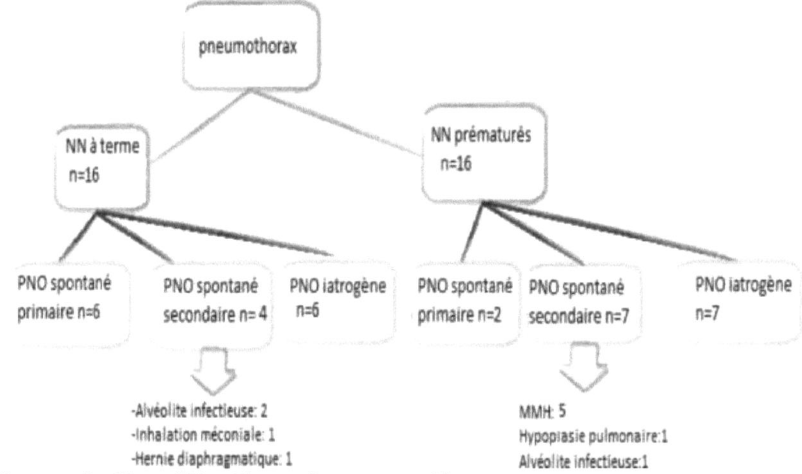

Figure 9: Classification of pneumothorax

-Iatrogenic PNO occurred in 40.6% of NN on artificial ventilation. NN were on CPAP in 15.6% of cases and on mechanical ventilation in 25%.

II. Topography of pneumothorax :

The PNO was unilateral in 75% of cases, with a right propensity in 20 NN.

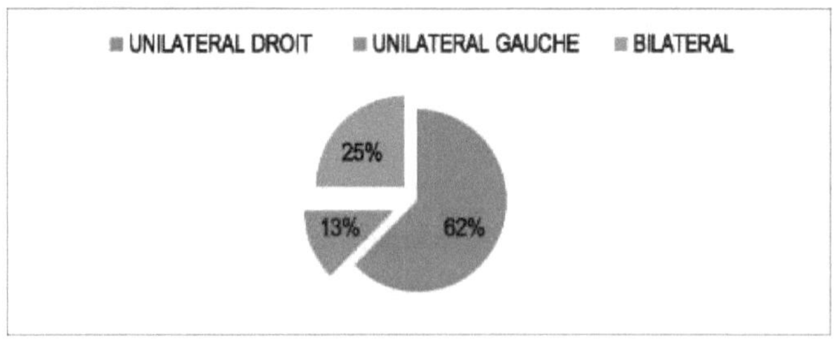

Figure 10: Topography of pneumothorax

ili. Pathologies associated with pneumothorax :

More than two-thirds of patients had a pathology associated with PNO on admission.

The respiratory pathologies associated with PNO MMH, infectious alveolitis and PAH. Lung hypoplasia was present as part of a Potter sequence in one case, and associated with a diaphragmatic hernia in another NN.

MFI was probable in 7 NN on the basis of anamnestic, clinical and biological criteria .

We have no bacteriological data to confirm this.

Fig. 10 summarises the various pathologies associated with PNO.

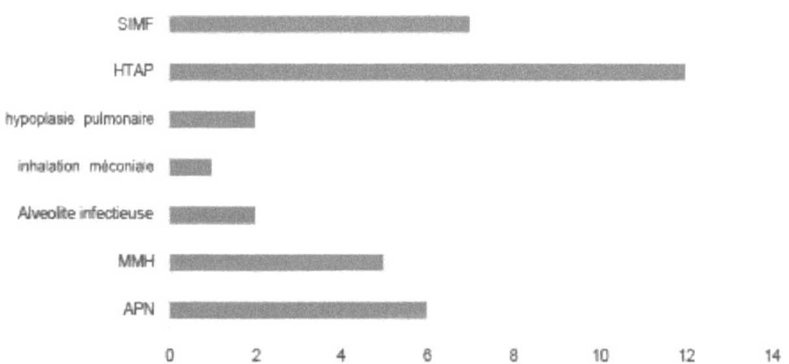

Figure 11: Pathologies associated with pneumothorax on admission

During their hospitalisation, NN presented with several comorbidities. Transfontanal ultrasound was only performed in NN in our study if neurological signs were present.

Figure 12 summarises the different pathologies presented by NN during hospitalisation

Figure 12: Comorbidities associated with pneumothorax occurring during hospitalisation

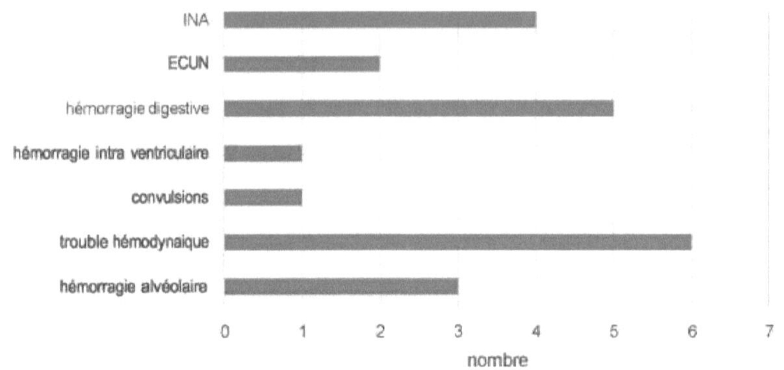

IV. MANAGEMENT OF PNEUMOTHORAX Management of pneumothorax

IV.1 Initial therapies (other than ventilation)

The initial management [the first 6 hours] of these NN consisted of conditioning them and using one or more of the drugs summarised in Table IV.

Table IV: Initial patient management

		Number	%
Medication	ATB *	25	21,8
	Surfactant	5	15,6
	Caffeine	9	28,12
	Tonicardiacs	6	18,7
Vascular approach	Peripheral venous access	25	21,8
	KTVO	5	15,6
	KTJ	2	6,2

*A maternal-fetal combination of betalactam antibiotics and single-dose or meningeal aminoglycosides was used, depending on the severity of the initial clinical picture. Surfactant instillation preceded the onset of PNO in 4 cases. The mean time between surfactant instillation and the onset of PNO was 110 min.

IV.2 Management of pneumothorax :

A wait-and-see attitude and hyperoxia (Fio2 at 100%) with close clinical and radiological monitoring was adopted in 7 cases. This attitude was adopted in 5 full-term babies and 2 near-term babies (35 and 36 SA). Exsufflation was performed in 23 cases (71.8%), followed by drainage in 15 cases. Drainage was performed immediately in 3 cases in the case of abundant pneumothorax that was not suffocating and when the patient's condition allowed it.

A rate of 62% required mechanical ventilation in "intermittent controlled assisted ventilation" (ICACV) mode (50%) or in "high frequency oscillation" (HFO) mode (12%).

Figure 13 below summarises the management procedures following the occurrence of a PNO.

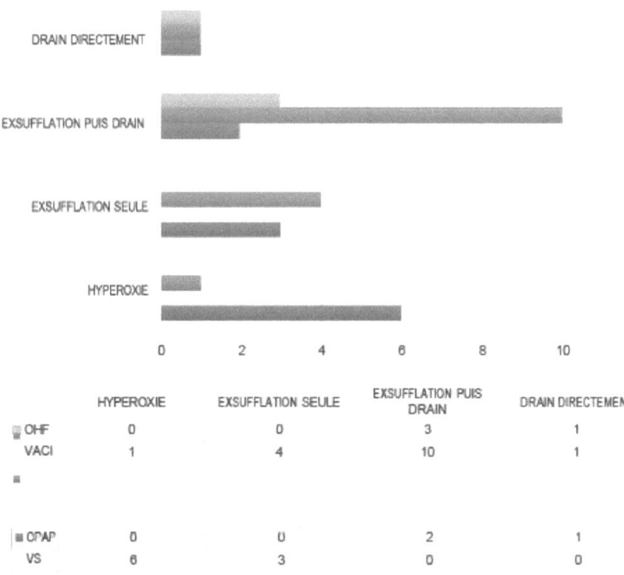

	HYPEROXIE	EXSUFFLATION SEULE	EXSUFFLATION PUIS DRAIN	DRAIN DIRECTEMEN
OHF	0	0	3	1
VACI	1	4	10	1
CPAP	0	0	2	1
VS	6	3	0	0

Figure 13: Management of pneumothorax

The absence of a mechanical ventilation machine in 2 cases led to CPAP with hyperoxia after exsufflation and drainage.

In 25% of cases, nitric oxide was administered mainly during the onset of PAH.

Figure 14 explains the circumstances in which each case of PNO occurs and how it is managed.

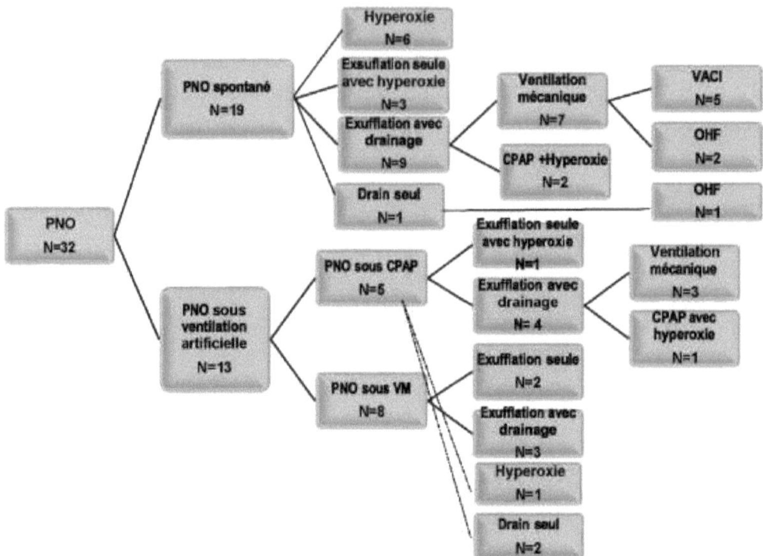

Figure 14: Management of pneumothorax according to the circumstances in which it occurs

V. Evolution of pneumothorax :

The PNO resolved in 65.6% of cases. In half the cases, resorption took place after 24 hours. The PNO worsened in 11 cases. Death from any cause occurred in 17 cases (53.12%). Death was attributed to the PNO in 2 cases: two cases of immediately suffocating PNO that did not respond to treatment, and in the other 2 cases the unavailability of a machine for mechanical ventilation was the cause.

The mortality rate in our study was high at 53.1%. The causes are summarised in Figure 15

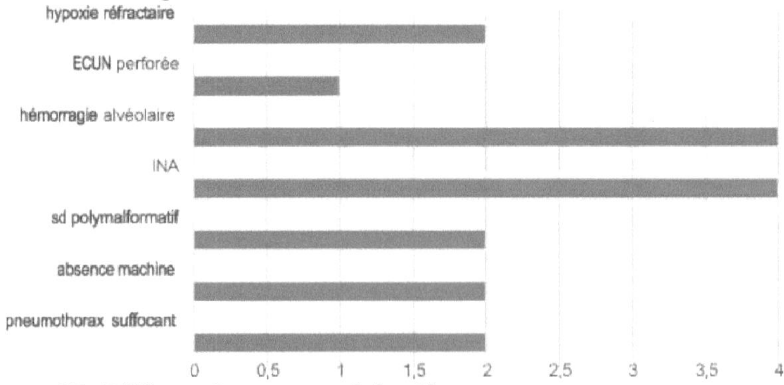

Figure 15: Different causes of death

C. Analysis of risk factors for pneumothorax :

1. Witness characteristics :

1.1 Maternal characteristics :

- **. Maternal age**

The average maternal age was 30.5 years, with extremes of 19 and 44 years. Mothers aged over 35 accounted for 17.2% of cases.

- **i. Characteristics of pregnancy and childbirth :**
- Pregnancy was spontaneous in 95.3% of cases
- Pregnancy monitoring was deemed to be compliant in 90.6% of cases.
- 4 cases of multiple pregnancy were recorded.
- 17.2% of mothers were toxemic; 25% had developed gestational diabetes during pregnancy
- Breech presentation was noted in 4 newborns (6.4%).
- 29.7% of pregnancies were complicated by a PMR>18h
- Delivery was complicated by acute fretal distress in 23 newborns, a rate of 35.9%. A cord circular was noted in 3 cases (4.9%).
- 4 cases of placenta previa (6.3%) and 4 cases of retroplacental haematoma were reported.
- Amniotic fluid was normal in 60 newborns, a rate of 93.8%. Oligohydramnios was noted in 3.1% of cases. Two cases of hydramnios were reported.
- The caesarean section rate (hot and cold) was 42.2%. Caesarean section was elective in 12 newborns, i.e. 44% of all caesarean sections.
- Instrumental delivery using Forceps was used in 3 deliveries; Figure 16 summarises the modalities in the control population

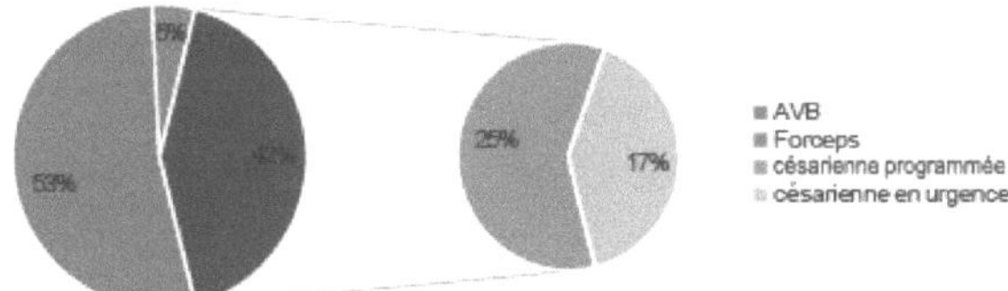

Figure 16: Delivery methods in the control population

- Meconium amniotic fluid was found in two newborns, and 6 cases of stained amniotic fluid were counted, representing 9.4% of newborns.

1.2 Characteristics of newborn babies :

i. Gender :

Our sample of control children was predominantly male, with an male, with a sex ratio (M/F) of 1.9 (Figure 17)

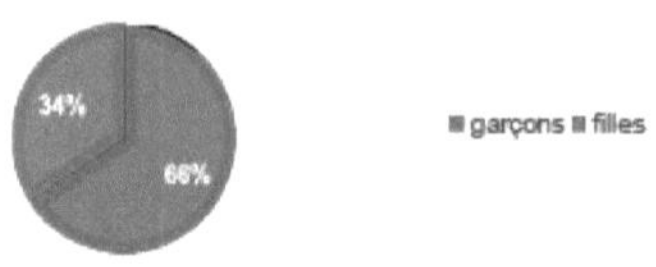

Figure 17: Breakdown of the control population by gender

ii. Birth weight :

The average birth weight was 2280g, with a minimum of 880g and a maximum of 4200g. The very low birth weight population represented 20.3% of the study population (Figure 18).

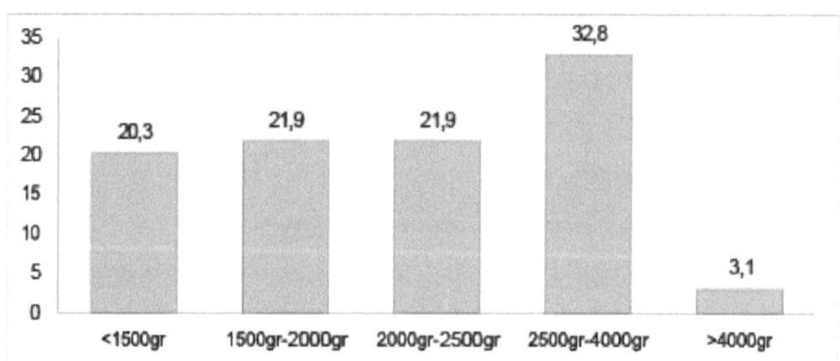

Figure 18: Distribution of the control population by birth weight

iii. Gestational age :

- The mean GA in our series was 35.7 SA with extremes ranging from 27 to 41 SA.
- Seventy-five per cent of the newborns were premature premature (GA < 37 SA), 33% of whom were very premature.
- No newborns were born post-term (GA> 42 SA)

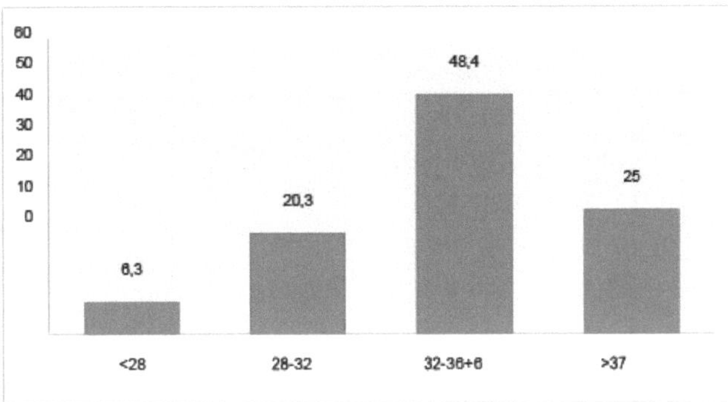

Figure 19: Distribution of control population by gestational age

iv. Condition of newborn babies in the delivery room :

- Seven children were born in a state of apparent death (table
- Mask ventilation at birth was used in

20.3% of NN and 15.6% were intubated in the
(Table V)

Table V:APGAR score of control patients

	Number	Frequency
Score at 1 min< 3	7	10,9
Score at 5min< 7	7	10,9

I.3 Characteristics of respiratory distress in the control population :

- The median Silverman score (SS) was 4 with extremes from zero to 6; signs of struggle were marked in 16 newborns, with a SS >4 . The SS was minimal between 0 and 1 in 6 newborns, i.e. 3.9% of cases.
- DRT followed by infectious alveolitis were the 2 most frequent etiologies of DRNN in the control population.
- During the first 24 days of life, 28 newborns (18%) were on CPAP; 3 on VACI (3.9%) and 5 on OHF (3.2%).

11. Risk factors for pneumothorax :

- The clinical characteristics of newborns who had had a PNO were comparable point by point to those of control children particularly for sex, gestational age and weight.
- Demographic data and comparative characteristics of all neonates are

presented in Table VI.

z Maternal data and the course of pregnancy and delivery in the two groups did not differ, except for oligohydramnios, which was significantly more common in the study population (p=0.039).

^ Patients born by caesarean section had a greater tendency to PNO, but without reaching a statically significant threshold (p=0.06). On the other hand, elective caesareans were more likely to develop PNO with p=0.04.

J Among resuscitation manoeuvres in the room, only mask ventilation is associated with a greater risk of PNO (p=0.03)

J There was a clear male predominance in both groups.

J Apgar scores at 1 and 5 minutes were not significantly different.

J Term newborns and those with a birth weight between 2500 and 4000g had a significantly higher risk of developing PNO during the first 24 hours of life, with p=0.014 and p=0.028 respectively.

J The MFI was not statistically significant in neonates with PNO. The unavailability of bacteriological samples in the majority of cases rendered this parameter uninterpretable.

J VACI was an important risk factor for the occurrence of PNO during the first 24 days of life, with a p=0.001

J Death was statistically more significant in the PNO population.

The factors most incriminated in the occurrence of death were : Cyanosis, suffocating PNO, association with haemodynamic disorders, occurrence on an MMH, the significance threshold if p<0.05.

Table VI: Demographic data and characteristics of newborns: case/control comparison

	Cases (n=32)	Controls (n=64)	Value of p
Average maternal age	31,7	30,5	0,33
Pregnancy follow-up	28	58	0,63
Oligohydramnios	5	2	0,039
Delivery route :			
-AVB	13	37	0,81
-Forceps	1	3	0,71
-Caesarean section (total)	19	27	0,06
-Elective caesarean section	12	12	0,04
Male sex	20	42	0,7
Gestational age (SA)			
>37	16	16	0,014
32-36+6	12	31	0,31
28-32	4	13	0,34
<28	0	4	0,14
Birth weight :			

>4000g	1	2	1
2500-4000g	18	21	0,028
2000-2499g	4	14	0,4
1500-1999g	4	14	0,4
<1500g	5	13	0,78
Apgar score at 1min<3	2	7	0 ,45
Apgar score at 5min<7	6	7	0,29
Meconium fluid	1	2	1
Resuscitation at birth :			
Free O2	27	55	0,92
Mask ventilation	12(37,5%)	13 (25,4%)	0,03
Intubation	8	10	0,26
VACI	8	3	0,001

4 DISCUSSION

The incidence of neonatal PNO and the risk factors favouring it have been the subject of few studies worldwide in general and in Tunisia in particular.

The results of our work show that pneumothorax is a common pathology in neonatal intensive care units and suggest the presence of associated risk factors. Therapeutic management varies. Mortality remains high despite advances in therapeutic methods. This calls for nationwide studies to determine the prevalence of PNO in Tunisia and to develop algorithms for its management.

The strong points of this work areon the one hand, the type of case-control study used to identify the risk factors for PNO, and on the other hand, it is the first study on Pneumothorax during the first 24 hours of life carried out at the Tunis Maternity and Neonatology Centre and, to our knowledge, in Tunisia.

The weaknesses of our study could be its retrospective nature, which explains the limitations encountered in the use of the data; the exclusion of newborns whose delivery occurred outside the maternity centre; and the absence of bacteriological data maternal-fetal infection.

A. CHARACTERISTICS OF THE STUDY POPULATION

I. Global data

Numerous studies have looked at pneumothorax in the general population, but few data have been published on the paediatric population.

Pneumothorax occurs in children during the neonatal period more than at any other time; it is a pathology frequently encountered in neonatal intensive care and occurs in 1-2% of newborns [1-2]. PNO can be iatrogenic or even occur spontaneously from the first breath and is due to a sudden increase in intra pulmonary pressure at birth leading to rupture of the alveolar membrane and penetration of air into the pleural space [2].

The incidence of pneumothorax is highly variable, depending on several factors;

Spontaneous pneumothorax occurs in 1-2% of term newborns and 6% of premature babies [3].

The incidence of PNO in mechanically ventilated premature newborns varies from 6 to 33% [2-5].
In a study conducted in Oman, the incidence of neonatal PNO 2.5/1000 births compared with 10-15/1000 in Denmark, 20/1000 in Turkey and 6.3/1000 in the Vermont oxford group [6].
Through a retrospective study over a period from 1st January 2014 to
On 31 December 2015, 378 NN were admitted to the neonatology and neonatal resuscitation department of Bega- Romanie among 4891 births. 12 cases of pneumothorax were noted, i.e. an incidence of 2.38% per year and a prevalence of 0.24% [7]
In a study by Zanardo et al. in Italy over a period of 2 years (2002-2003), 59 newborns were diagnosed with pneumothorax, i.e. 0.8/1000 births [8].
In a national multicentre study conducted in Malaysia, of 10387 newborn babies admitted to intensive care units, 505 developed pneumothorax, i.e. 4.9% of all gestational ages. [9]
In Korea, out of 4,414 newborns admitted to an intensive care unit, 57 patients had a PNO: 35 were at term and 22 premature, representing an incidence of 1.3% [10].
In Saudi Arabia, a recent study was carried out in a neonatal intensive care unit over a period of 3 years. 2204 NN were admitted. 86 patients had presented with PNO, an incidence of 3.9%. [11]
In our study, the incidence of pneumothorax occurring during the first 24 hours of life was 1.1/1000 births.
To our knowledge, no other published Tunisian study has investigated the prevalence of neonatal pneumothorax.

II. Maternal characteristics, pregnancy and childbirth :

Few studies have examined the relationship between neonatal PNO and maternal characteristics and the course of pregnancy and childbirth.
In a case-control study carried out in Thailand to determine the risk factors for PNO during the first 24 months of life, the average maternal age was 27.7 years. Pregnancy was correctly monitored in 82.5% of mothers. It was complicated by oligohydramnios in 3 cases (6.8%). Newborns born in pregnancies that were poorly or not monitored, or in cases of oligohydramnios, were at greater risk of developing PNO

(p=0.048 and p=0.04 respectively) [12].
In Malaysia, a national multicentre study was conducted to determine the risk factors for the occurrence of PNO in neonatal intensive care units. There were no significant differences associated with maternal age, gestational diabetes or multiple pregnancies. [9]
In a study carried out in Korea, among 35 term newborns with PNO, 28.6% had meconium fluid, 5.7% had RPM and 11.4% had perinatal asphyxia [10].
In our study, the mean maternal age was 31.7 years. A higher risk of pneumothorax was noted in the presence of oligohydramnios.
With regard to the route of delivery, all the data in the literature have confirmed the impact of caesarean section on neonatal respiratory morbidity.
Published studies show a higher incidence of pneumothorax in caesarean births (60-70%) [7-9, 13-16].
In the Bega-Romanie study, 90% of cases of pneumothorax were born by caesarean section and only 10% by vaginal delivery [7].
In Italy, Zanardo V studied the influence of the timing of elective caesarean sections on the occurrence of PNO. The incidence of PNO in cases of elective caesarean section, emergency caesarean section or vaginal caesarean section was 2.9/1000, 1.53/1000 and 0.39/1000 respectively [8].
In France, Girard I. studied the risk factors for pneumothorax in term newborns with neonatal respiratory distress. 96 NN were included over a 4-year study period, 32 of whom had a PNO. 45 (46.9%) were born by caesarean section, 30
(31.3%) by scheduled caesarean section at a median term for the latter of 37.9 SA [13].
A study conducted at Norway Oslo from 2001 to 2005 confirms that the incidence of PNO in caesarean sections is significantly higher than in vaginal deliveries (0.55 vs 0.10%; $p<0.001$) [15].
In our study, caesarean delivery tended to be associated with a higher risk of developing PNO without reaching a statistically significant threshold (p=0.06). This may be linked to the frequent use of caesarean sections in the 2 study groups. The practice of cold caesareans was preponderant in the group with PNO

III. Characteristics of newborn babies

III.1 Sex ratio :

Both in our series and in foreign studies, the predominance of males was noted at up to 65-70% [8].in our series, the sex ratio was 1.6.

In a retrospective study carried out from 1 January 2004 to 31 December 2007 in the neonatology and neonatal intensive care unit of the University of Reims, France, 32 cases of neonatal respiratory distress were associated with PNO, 75% of which were male [13].

Another study carried out in a neonatal intensive care unit at the São João Hospital Centre, Porto, Portugal between 2003 and 2014 included all cases of PNO, 62.5% were male [17].

In a retrospective epidemiological study of neonatal PNO during the first 24 hours of life in Thailand between 2001 and 2004, 71% were boys [12].

In Norway, in a 5-year retrospective, the risk of PNO was greater in boys than in girls (0.35% vs. 0.19%; $p<0.01$) [15].

III.2 Birth weight :

In an original study conducted by Aly H. in the Department of Neonatology at the National Pediatric Medical Center in Washington over a 10-year period concerning

77 cases of neonatal pneumothorax, with an incidence of 0.27% in neonates weighing > 2500 g and 2.5% in those weighing < 2500 g. The onset of pneumothorax in the 1st group occurred earlier in the first hours of life (mean 5.5 hours) compared with the 2nd group (mean H34 hours). [3]

The BEGA study found that 2/3 of patients had a low birth weight, of which 33% were between 2000 and 2500 g. [7]

A study carried out for the national neonatal registry in Malaysia in 2006 involving 26 neonatal intensive care units in the country included 505 cases of PNO, 42% of newborns had a weight >2500 g. The incidence of PNO in the low birth weight group was 3.5% for the weight range 10011500 g, compared with 7.3% in those under 1000 g [9].

In contrast, in a study carried out in Turkey involving 30 cases of neonatal PNO, 23 NN (i.e. 77%) had a PN > 2000g[18].

In our series, 59.4% of cases had a PN >2500 g; 15.6% of low birthweight cases had a PN <1000g. The onset of PNO in NN with a normal PN (>2500) was earlier: all cases were present before H1 of life. If we consider that PNO occurs later in NN of low birth weight, and given that our study only concerns PNO during the first 24 hours of life, which means that NN who developed PNO in the following days were not included, this could explain the predominance in our study of PNO in NN of normal weight.

111.3 Gestational age :

From the point of view of gestational age, in the scientific literature, the first place is occupied by term and post-mature newborns; the percentage varies according to the studies between 44% and 83% [7].

In a Canadian cohort from 2005 to 2011, the incidence of PNO was higher in term newborns (6.7%), followed by very premature infants (SA<32) (4%). In the intermediate gestational age group, the incidence was lower (2.6%) [19].

This bimodal distribution of pneumothorax, with the highest rates in term newborns and intermediate rates in the very premature, was probably due to several factors including population selection, pathophysiological variability at extreme gestational ages, and clinical management [19].

These results are in line with those found in the multicentre study carried out in Malaysia, where the highest rate of PNO was found in term newborns (6.3%) followed by very premature infants <32 SA in whom the incidence of PNO was inversely proportional to gestational age (6.8% in <26SA; 5.8% for 27- 29SA and 3.4% for 30-32SA) [9].

Our results are partially consistent with those in the literature, given that full-term newborns were in first place in 50% of cases. Extremely premature babies came last with 12.5% of cases. It should be remembered that our study only looked at PNOs during the first 24 hours of life.

111.4 Apgar score :

A few studies have reported the impact of a low Apgar score on the occurrence of PNO.

In a case control study conducted in Thailand to identify the risk factors associated with PNO during the first 24 hours of life, a low Apgar score at 1 and 2 minutes was associated with a higher risk of PNO. This may be explained by the often more vigorous resuscitation of NN with a poor APGAR score. As a result, PNO should always be considered in any newborn in the delivery room who does not respond to good resuscitation or vasoactive drugs, or who suddenly worsens during resuscitation [12].

A case control study carried out in Portugal showed a statistically significant difference in the occurrence of PNO and a low Apgar score at 5th minutes of life ($p<0.001$). This is often linked to resuscitation at birth in these patients. [17]

In a case-control study carried out in Iran over a period of 18 months involving 121 mechanically ventilated premature newborns, 42 had a PNO and 79 were unaffected. The mean Apgar score at 5 minutes was respectively 6.45 ± 1.5 and 7.39 ± 1.89 (P=0.06). A low APGAR score at 5 minutes of life represented the only risk factor for the development of a PNO according to the authors [20].

In a study including 16 cases of neonatal PNO in Nis-Serbia, 81.25% of patients had an Apgar score at 1 min of less than 3; the outcome of these patients was fatal in 30.8%.

In our series, the Apgar score was comparable in the 2 groups and was not a particular risk factor.

B. CHARACTERISTICS OF PNEUMOTHORAX

I. Clinical diagnosis :

Pneumothorax occurs more frequently during the neonatal period than at any other age, and often becomes apparent in the first 3 days of life [10].

Newborns with pneumothorax may be asymptomatic. These infants present in 1%-2% of all newborns and are often under-diagnosed: most often it is a minimal unilateral PNO. In the majority of cases, NN who have developed a PNO are symptomatic, either immediately or with a sudden and progressive onset of respiratory distress, irritability and apnoea [12].

Tachypnoea is the main symptom found in several studies. It may be associated with cyanosis or pallor and desaturation. Rapid recognition of PNO and early treatment prevent complications associated with hypoxaemia and hypercapnia [10].

In our study, we were only interested in PNO occurring during first 24 hours of life. Half of the cases of PNO were diagnosed before H1 of life; polypnoea was almost always present; cyanosis was reported in 14

cases.
This is in line with what has been described in the literature. In the study carried out in Bangkok, Thailand, tachypnoea was the main symptom in 95.5% of cases. The onset of PNO was immediate after birth in 38.6%; 88.4% before H6 of life and 95.3% before 12 hours of life. [12]
Katar S et al [21] conducted a prospective study of symptomatic spontaneous PNO in neonatal intensive care units in Turkey. Over a period of 22 months, 11 cases were analysed. All patients had respiratory signs starting 5 to 30 minutes after birth. Eight patients had O2 saturation <90%.

II. Type of pneumothorax :

Pneumothorax can be either primary spontaneous or idiopathic when there is no underlying pathology and no cause is found; or secondary if it occurs in pathological lungs. It is said to be iatrogenic when it is due to a medical or surgical procedure [10, 11, 17].
Spontaneous pneumothorax at birth results from alveolar rupture secondary to an increase in pressure necessary for the expansion of the lungs at birth or to an unequal distribution of pressures in the different alveoli [22].
There are rare specific forms of spontaneous pneumothorax known as "Familial" which appear to be genetically encoded [22].
Girard I et al. Carried out a 4-year study on a population of full-term neonates hospitalised in the neonatal intensive care unit for respiratory distress before 48 hours of life, with aim of determining the risk factors for developing pneumothorax in this population. Ninety-six children were included, 32 of whom had a PNO. Twenty-four NOPs (75%) were spontaneous, 6 (18.8%) were diagnosed after ambient or Neopuff ventilation in the delivery room, 1 (3.1%) after non-invasive ventilation (CPAP), 1 (3.1%) after invasive ventilation [8].
In the Portuguese study, of the 80 cases of PNO, 34 (42.5%) were iatrogenic. Among the other patients, 40 were secondary to an underlying pulmonary pathology and 6 cases were idiopathic (7.5%). [17]
In the Korean study, among 35 term NN, 20% had spontaneous PNO and 80% had secondary PNO [10].
These rates are similar to those found in Arabia Saudia in a study including 86 cases of neonatal PNO where the aetiology was identified in

76.7% of cases it appeared to be idiopathic in 23.3%. [11]

In our study, 8 cases of primary spontaneous pneumothorax were noted, i.e. 25% of cases, 75% of which were newborns at term.

III. Topography of pneumothorax :

Our study found that in 2/3 of cases the PNO was unilateral on the right and bilateral in 25% of cases, which is in line with the data in the literature concerning the location of pneumothorax.

The tendency for pneumothorax to occur on the right side may be due to the uneven distribution of air during the first few breaths. Oxygen therapy has been used in all cases to increase the adsorption of free air in the pleural cavity [12].

In a study carried out in Porto -Portugal from 2003 to 2014 including 240 NN including 80 cases of PNO, a predominance of the right side was found (46.3%) with bilateral involvement in 10% of cases [17].

The Bega study found the same results, with unilateral involvement in around 80% of cases, 45% of which were on the right side [7].

IV. Associated malformations :

In our study, we noted 2 cases of PNO associated with congenital malformations: in one case a diaphragmatic hernia diagnosed antenatally and in the other a renal agenesis in the Potter sequence. No cases of heart disease were reported.

These associations have already been described in the literature. Epithelial-mesenchymal tissue abnormalities, such as altered type IV collagen development, may contribute to pulmonary hypoplasia and urinary tract abnormalities [10]. Diaphragmatic hernia prevents lung expansion and promotes the development of PNO. [17]

In a study carried out in Turkey over a period of 10 years, 62 cases diaphragmatic hernia were collected; 18% of cases were complicated by PNO [23].

In a study conducted in Korea over a period of 9 years, 2.7% of the PNO cases studied had a renal anomaly such as hydronephrosis and grade IV vesico-ureteral reflux [10].

The coexistence of spontaneous PNO and congenital renal malformations was found by Ashkenazi et al. in a study of 23 cases of neonatal PNO, all of which underwent abdominal ultrasound. Eight cases (35%) had renal involvement: 3 had a Potter sequence, 1 patient had polycystic kidney disease and 4 had obstructive uropathy. Based on these results, the authors recommend screening renal ultrasound for NN with spontaneous pneumothorax of undetermined aetiology [24].

In Saudi Arabia, Al Tawil et al. reported that 1.7% of NN with PNO had congenital anomalies of the urinary tract [25].

In a study carried out in Turkey, 18% of patients had associated renal pathology (hydronephrosis and grade 2 pyelocalic ectasia). This study also suggested an association with cardiac abnormalities (55% of cases) [21], which was also found in a case-control study conducted in France [64].

Portugal over a period of 11 years. Of the 80 patients with PNO included in this study, 13.8% had associated congenital heart disease and 11.3% had diaphragmatic hernia ($p<0.05$) [17].

V. Management of pneumothorax :

Few studies have attempted develop an optimal management protocol for neonatal pneumothorax. Indeed, the treatment of neonatal pneumothorax is not fully defined. Three approaches are commonly used in intensive care units. Simple monitoring with free oxygenation for asymptomatic, low-abundance pneumothorax (<20-25%) versus urgent active intervention such as needle aspiration and chest drainage for moderate to severe cases.

Hyperoxia (FiO_2=100%) reduces nitrogen levels in the blood and creates a nitrogen pressure gradient between the pleural cavity and the blood capillary network, allowing absorption of the gas and reattachment of the pleural layers [35]. However, it should be remembered that a FiO_2 of 100% oxygen can be harmful, particularly in premature newborns, such as retinopathy of prematurity and bronchopulmonary dysplasia [35].

Needle exsufflation is often a life-saving procedure to control the emergency and allow a chest tube to be placed under optimal conditions. Needle aspiration with 65 hyperoxia without chest drainage is also an option in cases of mild to moderate pneumothorax when the infant is haemodynamically stable.

In tension pneumothorax, the common therapeutic approach is to place a chest tube. In the latter cases, mechanical ventilation is often required. [2, 7, 11, 12].

Thoracic drainage remains an invasive procedure that can lead to serious complications, particularly in neonates given their small thorax and narrow intercostal space. Pulmonary lesions, phrenic nerve paralysis,

chylothorax and haemopericardium have been reported following thoracic drainage in NN with PNO [26-28].
The method for estimating PNO size described by Rheaet al. in adult patients is difficult to relate to children, particularly NN. Consequently, the estimation of the size of the PNO and the decision of the treatment method remain operator dependent. Nevertheless, a large quantity of air with deviation of the mediastinal structures and depression of the homolateral hemi diaphragm require drainage [23,42].
Litmanovitz et al. conducted a retrospective study over 13 years in neonatal intensive care units. The aim of the study was to compare 2 groups of mechanically ventilated patients with PNO: those treated by thoracic drainage
versus those who did not. Of the 136 NN with PNO, 101 (74%) had a chest tube. In the 2nd group, 14 had needle aspiration while 21 were placed on expectant care. Ventilatory parameters (FiO2 requirements, ventilatory pressure, blood gases) were better in the 2nd group. [29]
In the study carried out in Saudi Arabia, 39% of NN remained under surveillance only, while 55.8% had a chest drain and 4.7% had needle aspiration. [11]
In the Korean study, 57 cases of neonatal PNO were included. Seven patients had spontaneous PNO, 71.5% of whom required chest drainage and mechanical ventilation, and only one case of spontaneous PNO resolved with hyperoxia. Of those with secondary PNO (50 cases), 53.6% underwent chest drainage and 42.9% required mechanical ventilation [10].
Trevisanuto et al [30] reported on a series of 61 neonates with PNO, 36% of whom did not have a chest drain: 16% had needle aspiration and 20% conservative treatment.
In the study carried out in Thailand, treatment was essentially symptomatic, with oxygen therapy aimed at achieving saturation of between 95% and 98% via a hood in 97.7% of cases. Chest drainage was performed in 6 cases. [12]
In Portugal, in a study including 80 NN who had developed PNO, 71.3% required chest drainage. Needle aspiration was performed in 10 cases (12.5%) but 7 required subsequent chest drainage. [17]
In our series, the choice of treatment was made by the medical team present. The three therapeutic approaches described in the literature

were applied according to gestational term, associated pathologies and the severity of the clinical and radiological picture. Seven patients, all at term, received hyperoxia with a Fio2=100%. Complete resolution of the PNO was noted in most cases within 24 hours. In only one case was the outcome fatal due to refractory hypoxia. Needle exsufflation was used in most cases as a means of rescue before proceeding with chest drainage.

VI. Evolution and mortality :

The mortality rate from neonatal PNO remains high despite advances in neonatal resuscitation techniques.

In the national multicentre study carried out in Malaysia, half of the NN who developed PNO died. The mortality rate varied according to term and birth weight. The mortality rate was 75% in babies under 24 weeks' gestation, 68.6% in the 24-27 weeks' gestation group, 59.7% in the 27-29 weeks' gestation group, 50% in the 30-36 weeks' gestation group and 34.4% in full-term infants. Similarly, the lower the birth weight, the higher the mortality rates: 100% for infants weighing 500 g at birth with pneumothorax, 72.3% for infants weighing between 501 and 1000 g and 32.4% for infants weighing more than 2500 g at birth. [9]

In a recent Canadian cohort of 24 neonatal intensive care units, PNO was associated with higher mortality in very premature infants, but not in moderately premature or term newborn infants. [19]

In the Saudia Arabia study, approximately 29.1% of NN with PNO had a fatal outcome. This rate was higher in cases of prematurity, low birth weight, low Apgar score and alveolar haemorrhage [11].

In Turkey, a study involving 60 cases of neonatal PNO was carried out assess the impact of PNO size on mortality. Unlike in adults, there are no data in the literature assessing the prognostic value of the size of neonatal PNO. In this study, PNO size was calculated on anteroposterior chest films by measuring the diameter of the PNO in relation to that of the thoracic cavity. The overall mortality rate was 30%, with a 13-fold increased risk in cases of PNO > 20% [31].

In our series, the outcome was fatal in 53.1% of cases. Our results will serve as a basis for possible future research and contribute to the optimisation and development of strategies.

to improve the management of PNO in neonatal intensive care units and reduce morbidity and mortality

C. ANALYSIS OF RISK OF PNEUMOTHORAX NEONATAL

Several risk factors for PNO in the neonatal period have been described in the literature. There are those associated with the course of pregnancy and delivery (monitoring of pregnancy, oligohydramnios, meconium fluid, chorioamniotitis, route delivery, etc.).); those relating to the newborn (gestational age, birth weight, sex, Apgar score, associated malformations, etc.) and finally those relating to the management of newborns (resuscitation in the delivery room, positive pressure ventilation, etc.) [2,8, 11,12,13].

Among maternal factors, poor pregnancy monitoring and poor socio-economic conditions have been associated with a higher risk of neonatal PNO [2,12].

In a study carried out in Thailand comparing 2 groups of patients in order to identify factors associated with PNO during the first 24 hours of life, the risk was 3.5 times greater in the case of a poorly monitored pregnancy. Similarly, in this study, the risk was greater in the case of oligohydramnios [12].

As for the mode of delivery, many studies have shown that a caesarean birth is associated with higher respiratory morbidity. Caesarean sections can result in excess lung fluid, particularly outside labour, since compression of the fretal thorax during contractions leads to the loss of large volumes of lung fluid. This route delivery disrupts the physiological changes that enable the newborn to adapt to normal cardiorespiratory conditions (secretion of catecholamines and glucocorticoids, inducing reabsorption of pulmonary fluid, secretion of surfactant and pulmonary vasodilatation), which explains the greater respiratory morbidity following caesarean section. A sudden pressure difference at the time of delivery by caesarean section leads to rupture of the alveolar membrane, which is all the more fragile in the case of a premature newborn, causing air to enter the pleural space, leading to neonatal pneumothorax [2, 11, 15, 19, 32].

In a case control study carried out in a neonatal intensive care unit in France over a period of 4 years, including 96 term newborns with respiratory distress, 32 of whom had presented with a PNO, I. Girard et al. identified two risk factors for PNO: birth outside a level III maternity hospital (so-called "outborn" newborns) and birth outside labour. Comparing the 2 groups of newborns with and without pneumothorax, the caesarean section rates were similar in the 2 groups, whereas absence from labour was more frequent in the group with pneumothorax ($p<0.05$). These results highlight the importance of labour in preparing the lungs for extra-uterine life and in preventing PNO. Programmed caesarean section should be avoided unless there is a clear medical indication, and should only be performed after 39 weeks' gestation [13].

This is in line with what has already been described by Zanardo et al. in Italy. Cold caesarean section is more likely to cause pneumothorax than vaginal caesarean section (OR 7.95; 95% CI 4.4114.32) and emergency caesarean section (OR 4.21; 95% CI 2.048.74). On the other hand, the occurrence of PNO is relatively greater in the case of emergency caesarean section than in the case of vaginal delivery [8].

According to the international literature, the risk factors associated with the patient include male sex, low birth weight and extreme prematurity, a low Apgar score and the existence an underlying pulmonary pathology (transient neonatal respiratory distress, hyaline membrane disease, pulmonary hypoplasia, etc.).

All published studies have concluded that the risk of developing PNO is higher in boys [7, 8, 15].

The higher risk of developing PNO in premature babies is explained by the immaturity of the lungs due to a lack of surfactant and higher intra-alveolar pressure, which leads to air trapping in the alveoli from the first breaths, causing them to rupture[2].

It is also known that PNO increases in cases meconium inhalation: the incidence is 10 to 30% [12].

The risk of PNO also depends on how resuscitation is carried out in the delivery room; high-pressure mask ventilation favours its occurrence [11, 19].

The use of invasive ventilation was incriminated in the occurrence of PNO. This was described in a study carried out in 18 centres in Poland over seven years: the incidence of PNO was 7.2% in NN undergoing invasive ventilation and 3.6% in those undergoing non-invasive ventilation ($p<0.001$) [33].

In a study carried out in Serbia, Terzic.S et al. found that a FiO2 requirement > 0.4 during the first 12 hours of life and recourse to mechanical ventilation were predisposing to the occurrence of PNO ($p < 0.05$) [34].

In our series, the comparative study with the control group enabled us to identify a certain number of risk factors for neonatal PNO. The existence of oligohydramnios, elective caesarean section, mask ventilation and invasive ventilation with IACV are risk factors for the occurrence of pneumothorax. This risk is all the greater during the first 24 hours of life when full-term newborns are involved. In contrast to the literature, low birth weight, Apgar score and meconium inhalation were not particularly associated with PNO.

5 CONCLUSIONS

Pneumothorax (PNO) is a frequent pathology in the neonatal period. Mechanical accidents linked to a sudden variation in pressure within the airways are encouraged by the first cry, the delivery process and any respiratory resuscitation manoeuvre. This is a vital emergency and a major cause of neonatal morbidity and mortality.

To this end, we proposed to carry out a retrospective study conducted in the neonatal intensive care unit of the Tunis maternity and neonatal intensive care centre over a period of 24months from 1st November 2014 until 31 October 2016. This study enabled us to determine the incidence and risk factors for the occurrence of pneumothorax during the first 24 hours of life in newborns admitted to the neonatal intensive care unit and to assess the management modalities for this condition during the neonatal period. To our knowledge, this is the first study in Tunisia of PNO during the first 24 hours of life.

To carry out this study, we selected all newborns admitted to the neonatal intensive care unit of the Tunis Maternity and Neonatology Centre (CNMT) during the study period who had presented with a pneumothorax during the first 24 hours of life. Controls were randomly selected among newborns admitted to the department for respiratory distress and whose birth followed or preceded that of the cases studied.

We excluded neonates transferred postnatally whose delivery did not take place at the Tunis maternity and neonatology centre.

In the first section, we present the overall epidemiology of cases of PNO, in the second section we study the main risk factors, and in the final section we assess the management methods used.

A total of **32** cases of pneumothorax (PNO) and 64 controls were included. During the study period, 28,800 live births (NV) were registered at the maternity centre, including 5,540 admissions to the intensive care unit. The incidence of PNO occurring during the first 24 hours of life was 1.1/1000 births.

The average maternal age was 31.7 years; all pregnancies were spontaneous and follow-up was considered satisfactory in 87.5% of cases.

The mothers were toxaemic in 12.5% of cases and 21.9% had developed gestational diabetes during pregnancy.

Oligohydramnios was noted in 15.6% of cases. cases of hydramnios

were reported.
The caesarean section rate was 62.5%. Caesarean section was elective in 12 newborns, i.e. 60% of all caesarean sections and 37.5% of PNO cases.
The delivery was complicated by acute fretal distress in 6 newborns, a rate of 18.8%. A circular cord was noted in 9.4% of cases. Three cases of placenta previa were reported.
Analysis of the characteristics of the newborns demonstrated the male predominance described in the literature, with a sex ratio of 1.6. Half of the newborns were premature (GA < 37 SA), 25% of whom were very premature. The average weight was 2636 g and 40.6% of cases had a low birth weight (<2500 g).
Mask ventilation in the delivery room was used in 37.5% of cases.
Half the cases of PNO were diagnosed before H1 of life; the most frequently described signs were polypnoea, cyanosis and desaturation. Spontaneous PNO was diagnosed in 19 cases, eight of which were idiopathic.
With regard to topography, approximately 2/3 of the PNOs described in the literature are unilateral and straight, and 15 to 25% are bilateral, which is consistent with the results of our study. In 31.3% of cases, the PNO was suffocating from the outset.
The PNO was associated with a diaphragmatic hernia in one case and a renal malformation in another.
Treatment modalities varied and were closely linked to the severity of the PNO. Management of pneumothorax was based on monitoring with hyperoxia to increase air resorption in 21.8% of cases. Needle exsufflation was performed in 68.8% of cases and chest drainage was required in 56.3% of cases. Mechanical ventilation in "intermittent controlled assisted ventilation" (ICACV) mode (50%) or "high frequency oscillation" (HFO) mode (12%) was required in 62% of cases.
The outcome was fatal in 53.1% of cases. Premature babies were involved in 64.7% of cases . Death was directly attributable to the PNO in 2 cases.
The comparative study with the control group enabled us to identify a certain number of risk factors. Oligohydramnios, elective caesarean section, mask ventilation and IVAC were risk factors for neonatal pneumothorax. These results are consistent with the literature.

At the end of our study, we were able to identify a number of guidelines for reducing the incidence of PNO during the first 24 hours of life. Further national studies are needed to assess the prevalence of neonatal PNO and to develop general guidelines for its management.

We therefore recommend :

- Good pregnancy monitoring.
- As far as possible, elective caesarean sections should be avoided before 39 weeks' gestation.
- If neonatal resuscitation is necessary, it must be carried out carefully in accordance with international recommendations;
- Pneumothorax should be suspected in all cases of respiratory distress whatever the term, and intervene early.

6 REFERENCES

1. Yu, V. Y. H., Liew, S. W., Roberton, N. R. C. Pneumothorax in the newborn: changing pattern. Archives of Disease in Childhood. 1975;50:449.

2. Dordevicl I, Slavkovicl A, Slavkovic-Jovanovic2 M, Marjanovicl Z. Influence of risk factors on frequency and prognosis of neonatal pneumothorax, five year experience. Acta Medica Medianae. 2010;49(2):5-8.

3. Aly H, Massaro A, Acun C, Ozen M. Pneumothorax in the newborn: clinical presentation, risk factors and outcomes. The Journal of Maternal-Fetal & Neonatal Medicine. 2014;27(4):402-6.

4. Ogata ES, Gregory GA, Kitterman JA, et al. Pneumothorax in the respiratory distress syndrome: incidence and effect on vital signs, blood gases, and pH. Pediatrics. 1976;58:177-83.

5. Goldberg RN, Abdenour GE. Air leak syndrome: Intensive care of the fetus and neonate: Mosby- Yearbook; 1996:629-40.

6. Ali R, Ahmed S, Qadir M, Maheshwari P, Khan R. Pneumothoraces in a Neonatal Tertiary Care Unit: Case Series. Oman Med J. 2013;28(1):67-9.

7. Iacob D, Agoston-Vas AE, Grajdeanu M, Dima M, Enatescu I, et al. NEONATAL PNEUMOTHORAX IN THE -BEGA|| NEONATOLOGY CLINIC BETWEEN 2014-2015. JURNALUL PEDIATRULUI. 2016; 19:73-74

8. Zanardo V, Padovani E, Pittini C, Doglioni N, Ferrante A, Trevisanuto D. The influence of timing of elective cesarean section on risk of neonatal pneumothorax. J Pediatr. 2007;150- 252.

9. Boo N-Y, Cheah IG-S, for the Malaysian National Neonatal Registry. Risk factors associated with pneumothorax in Malaysian neonatal intensive care units. Journal of Paediatrics and Child Health. 2011;47(4):183-90.

10. Lim, M.D., Ho Kim, M.D., Jang Yong Jin, M.D., Young Lim Shin, M.D., Jae Ock Park, M.D., Chang Hwi Kim, M.D. Sung Shin Kim, M.D .Characteristics of Pneumothorax in a Neonatal Intensive Care Unit Ho Seop. J Korean Soc Neonatol.
2011;18:257-264

11. Al Matary A, Munshi H. Characteristics of Neonatal Pneumothorax in Saudi Arabia: Three Years' Experience. Oman Medical Journal.2017;32(2):135-139

12. Ngerncham S.MD, Kittiratsatcha P.MD, Pacharn P.MD. Risk Factors of Pneumothorax during the First24 Hours of Life. J Med Assoc Thai. 2005; 88(8): 135- 41
13. I. Girarda, C. Sommerb, S. Dahana, D. Mitancheza, P. Morville Respiratory distress in term neonates: what are the risk factors for developing a pneumothorax? Archives de Pédiatrie.2012;19:368-373
14. Steele RW, Metz JR, Bass JW, DuBois JJ. Pneumothorax and pneumomediatinum in the newborn. Radiology. 1971;98: 629-32.
15. Benterud T, Sandvik L, Lindemann R. Cesarean section is associated with more frequent pneumothorax and respiratory problems in the neonate. Acta Obstetricia et Gynecologica Scandinavia. 2009; 88(3):359-61.
16. Jobe AH. Increased pneumothorax with elective C-section. The Journal of Pediatrics. 2007;150(3):A2.
17. Silva ÍS, Flôr-de-Lima F, Rocha G, Alves I, Guimarães H. Pneumothorax in neonates: a level III Neonatal Intensive Care Unit experience. Journal of Pediatric and Neonatal Individualized Medicine (JPNIM). 2016;5(2):e050220.
18. B Apiliogullari, Gs Sunam, S Ceran and H Koc: Evaluation of Neonatal Pneumothorax. The Journal of International Medical Research. 2011; 39: 2436 - 2440
19. Duong HH, Mirea L, Shah PS, Yang J, Lee SK, Sankaran K. Pneumothorax in neonates: Trends, predictors and outcomes. J Neonatal Perinatal Med. 2014;7(1):29-38.
20. Zarkesh M, Momtazbakhsh M, Mojtabai H. Incidence and risk factors of pneumothorax in premature low birth weight infants under mechanical ventilation. Iranian Journal of Neonatology IJN. 2013 Oct 1;4(3):1-6.
21. Katar S, Devecioglu C, Kervancioglu M, Ulku" R. Symptomatic spontaneous pneumothorax in term newborns. Pediatr Surg Int. 2006;22(9):755-758
22. Amuchou Singh S, Amin H. Familial Spontaneous Pneumothorax in Neonates. Indian J Pediatr 2005; 72 (5): 445-447
23. Gürsoy M , Shew SB, Ronna G. Miller, Smith EB , Gomez MR , Jaksic T. Survival Predictors In Congenital Diaphragmatic Hernia: Multivariate Analysis Of a 10- Year Experience. Journal of Turgut Özal Medical Center 1997;4(2):225-229
24. Ashkenazi S, Merlob P, Stark H, Einstein B, Grunebaum M,Reisner SH.

Renal anomalies in neonates with spontaneous pneumothorax-incidence and evaluation. Int JPediatr Nephrol. 1983;4:25-27
25. Al Tawil K, Abu-Ekteish FM, Tamimi O, Al Hathal MM, Al Hathlol K, Abu Laimun
8. Symptomatic spontaneous pneumothorax in term newborn infants. Pediatr Pulmonol 2004;37:443-446.
26. Kumar SP, Belik J. Chylothorax: a complication of chest tube placement in a neonate. Crit Care Med. 1984;12(4):411-412
27. Quak J, Szatmari A, van den Anker J. Cardiac tamponade in a preterm neonate secondary to a chest tube. Acta Paediatr. 1993;82(5):490-491
28. Odita JC, Khan AS, Dincsoy M, Kayyali M, Masoud A, Ammari. A. Neonatal phrenic nerve paralysis resulting from intercostal drainage of pneumothorax. Pediatr Radiol. 1992;22(5):379- 381
29. Litmanovitz I, Carlo WA: Expectant management of pneumothorax in ventilated neonates. Pediatrics.2008;122: e975 - e979
30. Trevisanuto D, Doglioni N, Ferrarese P, Vedovato S, Cosmi E, Zanardo V. Neonatal pneumothorax: comparison between neonatal transfers and inborn infants. J Perinat Med. 2005;33(5):449-454
31. Oze EA, Ergin AY, Sutcuoglu S, Ozturk C, Yurtseven A. Is Pneumothorax Size on Chest X-Ray a Predictor of Neonatal Mortality? . Iranian Journal of Pediatrics. 2013; 23 (5): 541-545.
32. Kamath BD, todd JK, GLazner JE. Neonatal outcomes after elective cesarean delivery. Obstet Gynecol. 2009; 113(6):1231
33. Wilinska M, Bachman T, Swietlinski J, Wilinski G. Pneumothorax in Neonates during Respiratory Support: Incidence, Timing, and Association with Mortality and Invasive Ventilation. Journal of Pediatric Sciences. 2014;6:e208
34. Terzic S, Heljic S, Panic J, Sadikovic M, Maksic H. Pneumothorax in premature infants with respiratory distress syndrome: focus on risk factors. Journal of Pediatric and Neonatal Individualized Medicine. 2016;5(1):e050124
35. Arda 4rfan Serdar, Gürakan B, APIefendioglu D, Tüzün M. Treatment of pneumothorax in newborns: Use of venous catheter versus chest tube. Pediatrics International. 2002 Feb 1;44(1):78-82.
36. Ogata ES, Gregory GA, Kitterman JA, Phibbs RH, Tooley WH. Pneumothorax in the respiratory distress syndrome: incidence and effect

on vital signs, blood gases, and pH. Pediatrics. 1976;58(2):177-183
37. Gibson C, Fonkalsrud EW. Iatrogenic pneumothorax and mortality in congenital diaphragmatic hernia. Journal of Pediatric Surgery. 1983;18(5):555-9.
38. Bashour BN, Balfe JW. Urinary tract anomalies in neonates with spontaneous pneumothorax and/or pneumonediastrnum. Pediatrics 1977;59:1048-9.
41. A. K. Mandal, S. Yamini, and X. Bean. Arterial blood gas and expiratory pressure monitoring in infants with pneumothorax: prognostic predictability. J Natl Med Assoc. 1990; 82(1): 33-37.
42. Rhea JT, DeLuca SA, Greene RE. Determining the size of pneumothorax in the upright patient. Radiology 1982; 144:7336.
43. Ramesh Bhat Y, Ramdas V. Predisposing factors, incidence and mortality of pneumothorax in neonates. Minerva Pediatr. 2013;65(4):383-8.

7 APPENDICES

APPENDIX 1: Study sheet

Newborn: -Identity : Tel

- gender: Mo Fo

-Date of birth :

Maternal features :

Age : <20y □ 20-35□ >35- **Blood type:**

Consanguinity: yes □ no □ ;

G..../P....EV....

Characteristics of the current pregnancy :

Correct monitoring of pregnancy* : yes-no ; **Normal ultrasound** : our-no ; if No :

Spontaneous pregnancy: yes-no ;

Multiple pregnancies: yes-no

Pregnancy complications

- **Oligohydramnios**: yes-no; - **hydramnios**: yes-no;

Placena pravea: yes-no

- **CFS (IUGR)**: yes-no; - **Fetal-pelvic disproportion**: yes-no;
- **TG**: yes-no
- **DG**: yes-no ; **-Maternal hypothyroidism**: yes-no ;

MAP yes-no**; CAN**: yes-no

Circumstances of delivery

TIU : : yes- no **Location** : CHU- CHP - Ambulance -

At home ; **Presentation**: vertex- seat- bregma- forehead- face- shoulder

Appearance of amniotic fluid: clear- tinted- meconium- ;

SFA: yes-no; **Chorioamniotitis**: yes-no;

RPM>18h: yes-no; **Maternal fever**: yes-no;

Delivery route : * **AVB** or non-AVB: without intervention -

With intervention- Type of intervention: Episiotomy- vacuum- forceps- ***C/S** ori- no :

indication for caesarean section **Elective C/S**: yes' no' ;

C/S AG: yes' no' ; **C/S Peridural**: yes' no' ;

RSD: yes' no' **; O2 free**: yes' no' ;

Tracheal aspiration of meconium: yes' no' ;

VPP: yes' no'**; Intubation**: yes' no'; **Narcan:** yes' no'.

Characteristics of the study population

Gestational age : **<28** yes' no' **; 28-32** yes' no' **;**

32-36+6j: yes' no' **; 37-42:** yes' no' **; >42** yes' no' ;

Birth weight : **<1500** yes' no' ; **1500-2000** : yes' no' **;**

2000-2500: yes' no' ;

>2500 : yes' no'

Apgar score : 1min 5min 10min Reason for hospitalisation

Characteristics of the PNO

Date of occurrence : ; **H1:** yes' no' **; <H12**: yes' no' ; **H12-H24**: yes' no' ;

Severity*: **simple detachment**: yes' no' ;
moderate: yes' no'; **suffocating**: yes' no'.

Location: one-sided right: yes' no' ;
unilateral left: yes' no'; bilateral: yes' no'.

Circumstances of discovery: Incidental: yes' no' if yes: **X-ray:** yes' no'; **clinical:** yes' no'.

|**EMA**: yes' no' ;

Respiratory signs: yes' no' :
cyanosis yes' no' ;
signs of struggle yes' no' ;
isolated polypnoea: yes' no' ;

Desaturation: yes' no' ; **HRT**: yes' no' ;

Radiological appearance: Association: + +

1. Hyperclarity with disappearance of the lung parenchyma on the affected side yes' no'
2. Reduction or absence of pulmonary vascularisation . yes' no'
3. Increase in the volume of the affected hemithorax yes' no'
4. Enlargement of EICs.yes' no'.
5. Flattening of the diaphragmatic dome on the affected side . yes' no' .
6. Sharp edge sign. yes' no'
7. Deviation of mediastinum and/or heart and/or trachea with reduction in volume of healthy lung yes' no'
8. narrow cardiac silhouette . yes' no

Associated effusion: yes' no' : **PNM:** yes' no' ;

Hydrothorax: yes' no' ;

Pneumopericardium: yes' no'; **Subcutaneous emphysema**: yes' no'.

Management of the PNO

	O	N	Duration	VM	VM duration	**OTHER**	O	N	Duration
Oxygen-free preservative						Drug vaso A ~			
Oxygen to maintain correct saturation						Prostine			
Hyperoxia			-			sedation			
Exufflation , hyperoxia			-			filling			
Exufflation, CPAP			-			Corticoides			
Exufflation , drainage									
Exufflation , drainage , VM			-	-	-				
Nitrogen			-	-	-				

Monitoring

I R*thorax/24h I Number I

Plan before PNO	Yes	No				
Perfusion before PNO	Yes	No	VVP	KTVO	KTB	KTJ

Associated co-morbidities -Evolution of the PNO									
associated morbidities	**O**	**N**	**Date**	**Type**		**Evolution O**		**N**	**Type**
AI									
DRT									
MMH						In favour :Resolution			
HDC						<24H			
IM						24H-3d			
Congenital heart disease				-		>3j			
MFI						Worsening			
IAS						PAH			
PAH						Deaths			
Neurological . distress				-		**Cause of death**			
ECUN									
HD disorders						No machine			
Alveolar Hg						Suffocating from the start			
Kidney damage				-		Comorbidity			-
Surgical malformation				-					
DBP									

Additional tests: the first 24 hours
-Biology : *grouping : *NFS : *CRP :
* Blood culture: ... *Peripheral samples:...
*Haemostasis : *Blood glucose : *Ionogram /urée/creat
-O2 saturation : -Blood gas: *Po2 : *Pco2 : ETF
FO

APPENDIX 2: Thoracic exufflation

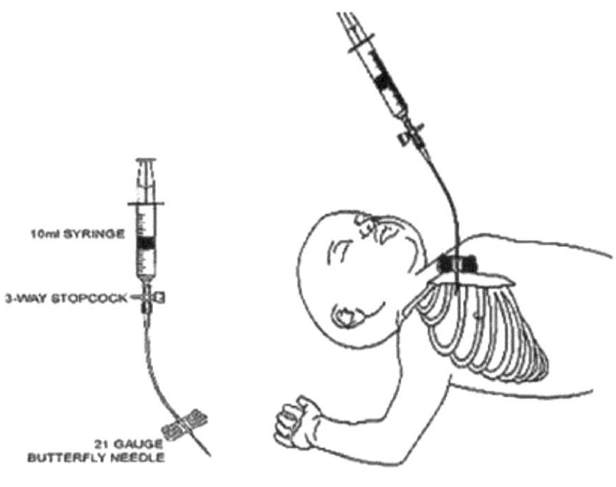

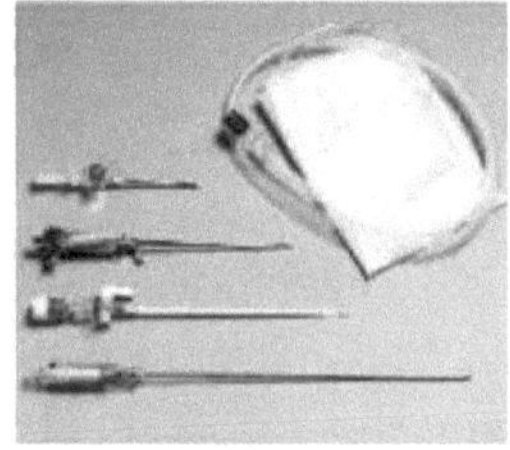

Exsufflation equipment (G 21 epicranial, three-way tap, 20 ml syringe)
Dressing material

Placing the pleural drain

Pre-analgesia xylocaine® ***Asepsis +++***

- The equipment

- a single-use drain-trocart, consisting of a metal mandrel with a pointed distal tip or a foam tip with a proximal tip fitted with a safety bulge. This mandrel fits exactly inside a transparent, perforated, graduated drain with an X-ray opaque rib (Joly drain, small - Mallinckrodt drain, large).
- a Drainopack®, or other equivalent material
- Installation
- disinfect the operating field, place the sterile drape
- Cutaneous incision with a scalpel, the size of the diameter of the drain, opposite the upper edge of the rib (3rd-4th IC space), at the level

of the middle axillary line .

- Insert the trocar perpendicularly to the wall, using one hand as a "fou||guard" to pull it back in as soon as the resistance gives way, indicating that the drain is in the pleural cavity. Remove the mandrel.
- push the drain into the pleural cavity towards the lower third of the sternum (where air collects in a child lying supine). Clamp it.
- close the skin wound with a knotted thread, passed around the drain in a spartan fashion to secure it to the skin.
- apply the dressing (see diagram)
- connect the declamped drain to the drainage system (figure).
- radio to check the position of the drain

2. Drainage monitoring

With the suction set to the desired vacuum (-15, -20 cm H2O), there is moderate bubbling in the control compartment. The patient is feeling better...

The drainage device must never be placed higher than the patient's thorax.

3. Removing the drain

- when the chest X-ray is satisfactory and the drain is llexclull (= no longer productive, no longer transmitting breathing-related oscillations).
- after disinfecting the skin, the surgeon cuts the thread attaching the drain to the wall and removes it; the skin is massaged to separate the different layers, and the wound is closed with a steristrip®.
- end of drain cultivated.
- radio control within a few hours.

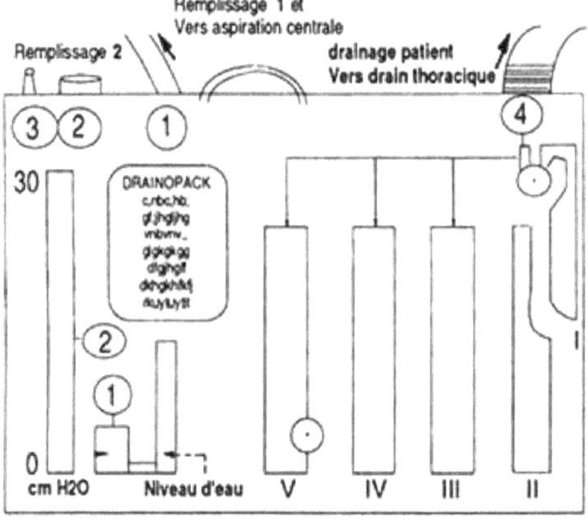

1) Filling chamber **1**: with a syringe filled with distilled water, connected to tube **1**, up to the water level (backflow prevention).

2) Vacuum adjustment: through opening **2**, fill chamber **2** to the required vacuum level (maximum 30 cm H2O).

To reduce the vacuum, connect a syringe to cone luer **3** and aspirate.

3) Connect the chest tube to tube **4**

4) Connect tube **1** to the central vacuum. Switch on the central suction and check that it is working correctly by observing bubbles in chambers **1** and **2**.

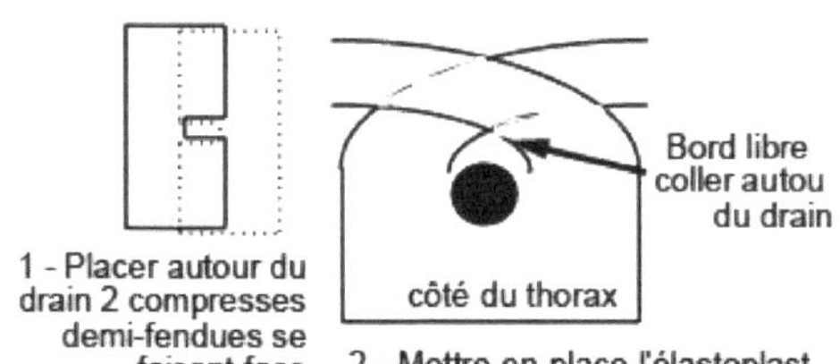

1 - Place 2 half-slit compresses around the drain, facing each other

Free edge glued around the drain

2 - Fitting the elastoplast

Pleural drain dressing

APPENDIX 4

! I. Infant Flow® SiPAP System

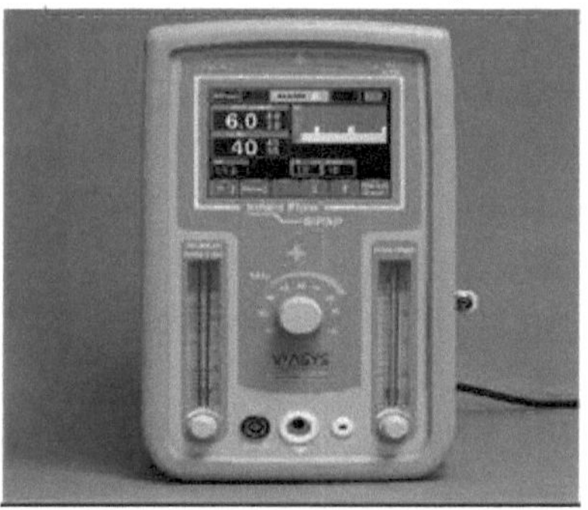

! II. Drager Babylog VN500

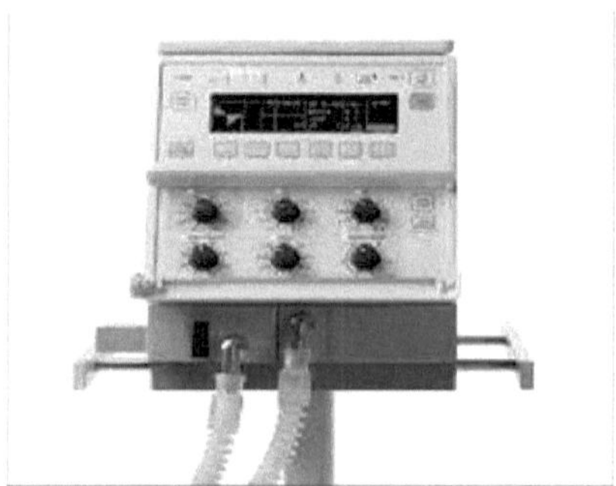

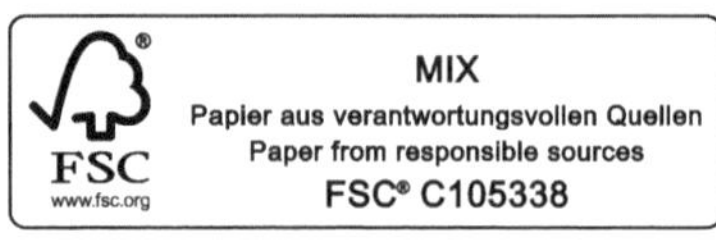

Printed by Books on Demand GmbH, Norderstedt / Germany